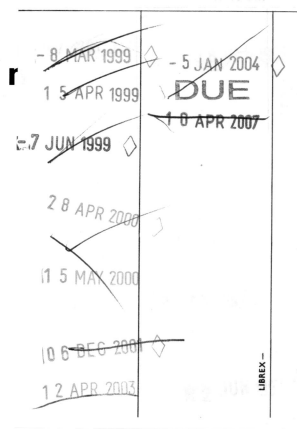

D
664.0288
SAF

World Health Organization
Geneva
1994

WHO Library Cataloguing in Publication Data

Safety and nutritional adequacy of irradiated food.

1. Food irradiation 2. Food preservation
3. Nutritive value

ISBN 92 4 156162 9   (NLM Classification: WA 710)

The World Health Organization welcomes requests for permission to reproduce or translate its publications, in part or in full. Applications and enquiries should be addressed to the Office of Publications, World Health Organization, Geneva, Switzerland, which will be glad to provide the latest information on any changes made to the text, plans for new editions, and reprints and translations already available.

© World Health Organization 1994

Publications of the World Health Organization enjoy copyright protection in accordance with the provisions of Protocol 2 of the Universal Copyright Convention. All rights reserved.

The designations employed and the presentation of the material in this publication do not imply the expression of any opinion whatsoever on the part of the Secretariat of the World Health Organization concerning the legal status of any country, territory, city or area or of its authorities, or concerning the delimitation of its frontiers or boundaries.

The mention of specific companies or of certain manufacturers' products does not imply that they are endorsed or recommended by the World Health Organization in preference to others of a similar nature that are not mentioned. Errors and omissions excepted, the names of proprietary products are distinguished by initial capital letters.

TYPESET IN INDIA
PRINTED IN ENGLAND

93/9707—Macmillan/Clays—7000

Contents

Preface	vii
Executive summary	ix
1. Introduction	1
References	3
2. Food irradiation	4
2.1 History of food preservation	4
2.2 Radiation sources	5
2.3 Mechanism of food irradiation	7
2.4 Activity in biological systems	9
2.5 Previous reviews	11
References	13
3. Applications	16
3.1 Introduction	16
3.2 Functions	17
3.3 Plant products	18
3.3.1 Fresh fruits and vegetables	18
3.3.2 Nuts and dried fruits and vegetables	22
3.3.3 Spices	22
3.3.4 Grains and grain products	23
3.4 Animal products	24
3.4.1 Poultry	24
3.4.2 Meat	24
3.4.3 Seafood	25
3.4.4 Eggs	27
3.4.5 Dairy products	27
3.5 Combination processes	27
3.6 Summary and conclusions	28
References	29

CONTENTS

4. Chemistry of food irradiation   35

    4.1 Introduction   35
    4.2 Background radiation and induced radioactivity   35
    4.3 Types of radiation and their effects   36
    4.4 Water   37
    4.5 Dilution   38
    4.6 Multicomponent systems   38
    4.7 Oxygen   38
    4.8 pH   39
    4.9 Temperature   39
    4.10 Radiolytic products   39
    4.11 Effects on major food constituents   39
        4.11.1 Carbohydrates   39
        4.11.2 Proteins   40
        4.11.3 Lipids   41
        4.11.4 Vitamins   42
        4.11.5 Conclusions   42
    4.12 Total yield of radiolytic products   43
    4.13 Unique radiolytic products   43
    4.14 Summary and conclusions   45
    References   45

5. Post-irradiation detection methods   50

    5.1 Introduction   50
    5.2 International activities   51
    5.3 Methods   52
        5.3.1 Chemical changes   52
        5.3.2 Physical properties   58
        5.3.3 Histological, morphological and biological effects   65
    5.4 Harmonization of protocols and testing strategies   66
    5.5 Summary and conclusions   67
    References   67

6. Toxicology   81

    6.1 Introduction   81
    6.2 Toxicity studies   82
        6.2.1 Studies in the FDA electronic database   82
        6.2.2 Raltech studies   102
        6.2.3 Human feeding studies in China   103
        6.2.4 Other studies   104
        6.2.5 International Project in the Field of Food Irradiation   105
    6.3 Summary and conclusions   106
    References   107

CONTENTS

7. Microbiology — 122

7.1 Introduction — 122
7.2 Selective killing and differential growth — 123
7.3 Mutations — 125
7.4 Mycotoxin production — 127
7.5 Summary and conclusions — 128
References — 128

8. Nutritional quality — 132

8.1 Introduction — 132
8.2 Synopsis of reviews — 133
    8.2.1 International reviews — 133
    8.2.2 National and regional reviews — 133
    8.2.3 Reviews by the scientific community — 134
    8.2.4 Conclusions — 135
8.3 Nutrient levels — 135
    8.3.1 Purpose of study — 135
    8.3.2 Radiation dose — 136
    8.3.3 Radiation source — 136
    8.3.4 Temperature — 136
    8.3.5 Hydration — 137
    8.3.6 Individual nutrients — 138
    8.3.7 Atmosphere at the time of irradiation — 141
    8.3.8 Storage conditions — 141
    8.3.9 Antimetabolites — 142
8.4 Role of irradiated food in the total daily diet — 143
8.5 Preregistration requirements — 143
8.6 Labelling — 143
8.7 Postmarketing surveillance — 144
8.8 Research needs — 144
8.9 Summary and conclusions — 144
References — 145

9. Concerns and overall conclusions — 149

9.1 Concerns expressed about irradiated food — 149
    9.1.1 Conflicting results and conclusions — 149
    9.1.2 Radiolytic substances — 149
    9.1.3 Fears of radioactive food — 149
    9.1.4 Dead food — 149
    9.1.5 Use of irradiation to restore contaminated food — 150
    9.1.6 Aflatoxin — 150
    9.1.7 Botulism — 150

CONTENTS

     9.1.8   Nutrients   151
     9.1.9   Resistant microorganisms   151
     9.1.10 Organoleptic effects   151
     9.1.11 Labelling   151
     9.1.12 Lack of adequate controls   152
     9.1.13 Dose uniformity   152
     9.1.14 Post-irradiation detection methodology   152
     9.1.15 Re-irradiation   152

9.2 Overall conclusions   153
References   153

Annex. Participants in WHO Consultation on Food Irradiation   154

Index   156

Preface

Food irradiation has, in certain circumstances, an important role to play both in promoting food safety and in reducing food losses. Because the safety and availability of nutritious food are essential components of primary health care, the World Health Organization is concerned that the unwarranted rejection of this process, often based on a lack of understanding of what food irradiation entails, may hamper its use in those countries likely to benefit most.

WHO actively encourages the proper use of food irradiation in the fight against foodborne diseases and food losses. To this end, it collaborates closely with Member States and other international organizations, particularly through the Joint FAO/IAEA/WHO International Consultative Group on Food Irradiation.

This up-to-date report on food irradiation has been produced at the request of one of WHO's Member States. Scientific studies carried out since 1980 have been reviewed and evaluated in its preparation, as have many of the older studies which had already been considered by previous international and national expert committees. Such controversial issues as the Indian studies on malnourished children fed freshly irradiated wheat (leading supposedly to a pathological condition, polyploidy) and the many claims that irradiation destroyed the nutritional value of food were given particular consideration[1] and were evaluated by a group of experts who, with one exception, had not previously been called upon by WHO to undertake the evaluation of irradiated food.

The first draft of the present publication was prepared by Dr Gary Flamm, with the help of Dr George Burdock, Dr Allan Forbes, Dr John Little, Dr Pasquale Lombardo and Dr Warren Nichols. Following a consultation[2] to review and revise the text held in Geneva from 20 to 22 May 1992, Dr Flamm prepared a provisional report, which was issued by WHO in October 1992 as an unpublished document (WHO/HPP/FOS/92.2) in a limited number.

---

[1] In the preparation of this report, the world's scientific literature was searched, electronically stored data were accessed and the contents of dockets and files at the Food and Drug Administration in the USA and the US Department of Agriculture, as well as the data stored in Karlsruhe, Germany at the Federal Research Centre for Nutrition, were reviewed.
[2] See Annex for a list of participants.

The present publication is the result of further review and refinement of the provisional report, taking into account in particular the comments of the observers from the National Food Authority of Australia and from the International Organization of Consumers Unions.

Executive summary

1. Applications

Food irradiation can have a number of beneficial effects, including delay of ripening and prevention of sprouting; control of insects, parasites, helminths, pathogenic and spoilage bacteria, moulds and yeasts; and sterilization, which enables commodities to be stored unrefrigerated for long periods.

The shelf-life of many fruits, vegetables and meats can be extended by irradiation. Sprouting in root crops such as potato, sweet potato, yam, turnip, carrot, onion, garlic, shallots, beets, and Jerusalem artichoke can be inhibited with irradiation doses of 0.05–0.15 kGy. Irradiation of tropical and sub-tropical fruits such as bananas, mangoes, papayas and guavas at doses of 0.25–1 kGy delays maturation and senescence. Ripening is suppressed in temperate-zone fruits such as apples, pears and stone fruits at doses in excess of 1 kGy, although this often results in some damage to the fruit. Mushrooms irradiated at doses up to 1 kGy may have their shelf-life extended by as much as 5–7 days. Strawberries are relatively resistant to damage by ionizing radiation, and irradiation at 2–2.5 kGy in combination with refrigeration can increase shelf-life by 1–2 weeks.

Levels of spoilage bacteria in poultry may be reduced sufficiently to prolong shelf-life by as much as 1–2 weeks following exposure at 3 kGy. Most of the spoilage organisms in meats can be killed by substerilizing doses of ionizing radiation, resulting in a significant extension of shelf-life. Many meats can tolerate relatively high doses of irradiation if appropriate precautions are taken. For example, blanching, freezing and the exclusion of oxygen together with doses in the 25–45 kGy range can result in sterilized food with a long shelf-life. Substerilizing doses of ionizing radiation can also extend the shelf-life of fish and shellfish.

Many important fresh fruit and vegetable pests, including fruit flies, the mango seed weevil, the navel orange worm, the potato tuber worm, the codling moth, spider mites and scale insects, may be controlled by doses of 1 kGy or less. Insect disinfestation of nuts and dried fruits can also be achieved, since most insects are killed by doses in the range 0.25–0.75 kGy.

Spices and related materials may contain large amounts of moulds, bacteria, and their heat-resistant spores. Doses of 3–10 kGy can significantly improve the hygienic quality of spices, dehydrated vegetables, herbs, and other dry ingredients. Doses of 1 kGy or less can prevent losses from insect infestation in stored grains, pulses, flour, cereals, and coffee beans.

Much of the raw poultry sold for human consumption is contaminated with *Salmonella* and *Campylobacter,* both of which can be effectively controlled by irradiation, as they are readily destroyed by doses in the range 2–3 kGy. Irradiation of pork at doses of 0.3 kGy or less can kill the larvae of the parasite *Trichinella spiralis*, and low-dose irradiation may also reduce the risk of cysticercosis caused by the pork tapeworm. Infections resulting from the consumption of undercooked beef containing beef tapeworm cysts may be prevented by irradiation at a minimum dose of 0.4 kGy.

It is most unlikely that all these potential applications will prove commercially acceptable; the extent to which such acceptance is eventually achieved will be determined by practical and economic considerations.

2. Chemistry

There are many forms of radiation, but only high-energy radiation can produce ions or charged particles after being absorbed by matter. This type of radiation is called ionizing radiation, and comprises gamma rays from decaying radioisotopes, X-rays, and machine-generated electrons. Absorption of ionizing radiation by food molecules results in the breaking of chemical bonds and the generation of free radicals and charged ions, leading to the formation of radiolytic products. The study of the chemistry of food irradiation has largely focused on the nature of these products.

Each of the three major macronutrients in food—carbohydrates, proteins and lipids—gives rise to different types of radiolytic products when exposed to ionizing radiation. Water plays a key role in influencing the nature and yield of the products from carbohydrates which, in the presence of water, react chiefly with hydroxyl radicals, producing ketones, aldehydes and acids. Sugars are also formed from starches. Amino acids undergo reactions including abstraction of hydrogen, reductive deamination, disproportionation, decarboxylation, and reaction of intermediates with the highly reactive products of water radiolysis. When proteins are irradiated in the presence of water, all the reactions that amino acids undergo may also take place in proteins containing these amino acids. As a result, large numbers of different radiolytic products may be formed. Degradation of proteins to smaller polypeptides may occur, but aggregation of proteins is also possible. In a food matrix, the amino acids contained in a protein are much less subject to attack than in pure solution because they are relatively inaccessible. In contrast to carbohydrates and proteins, the irradiation chemistry of lipids does not involve water, as they are virtually insoluble. A wide range of radiolytic products may be formed, including fatty acids, esters and diesters, aldehydes, ketones, alkanes and alkenes, diglycerides and shorter-chain triglycerides. In a meat matrix, oxidative changes in lipids are relatively minor because of possible antioxidant effects of proteins with increasing radiation dose. It is important to emphasize that, while a wide range of radiolytic products may be formed in the three major macronutrients, with good manufacturing practice radiation affects less than 1–2% of the macronutrients in food.

The study of the chemistry of the effects of irradiation on vitamins has focused chiefly on the extent of nutrient loss. In pure solution, vitamin destruction is far greater than that observed in foods. With some exceptions, the destruction of vitamins caused by the irradiation of food is relatively small, resulting in little change in overall nutritional value. The extent to which vitamins are lost through irradiation depends on both food type and storage conditions.

There has been much discussion over whether irradiation of foods produces unique radiolytic products, i.e. compounds not found in foods either in the natural state or as a result of conventional food processing. As it will be difficult to establish that such products exist, concern about their toxicological potential is speculative.

The United States Army has produced detailed analyses of 65 volatile chemicals in irradiated beef. Also in the United States, the Food and Drug Administration (FDA) reported that six of these chemicals could not be identified in volatile fractions of nonirradiated foods, and therefore suggested that they might be unique. Further investigation showed that only three of the six (undecyne, pentadecadiene, and hexadecadiene) had not been found in non-irradiated foods. These chemicals are not unusual; compounds differing from them by only one carbon atom have been detected in nonirradiated foods. The existence of such very close homologues suggests that the three apparently unique radiolytic products probably exist at some level in non-irradiated foods, and might be found if more sensitive analytical techniques were to become available. In the same way, more sensitive analytical techniques might eventually reveal the existence of unique radiolytic products at extremely low levels.

The example cited above concerns reaction products associated with a volatile fraction, and this is probably typical of the relationship of nonvolatile radiolytic products and possibly of unique radiolytic products to one another, and to radiolytic products that are constituents of nonirradiated foods. Whether radiolytic products are unique or not, enzymatic hydrolysis would be expected to transform most of them into common compounds, such as fatty acids, amino acids, monosaccharides, and other products resulting from the human digestive process.

All foods are to some extent radioactive, generally at extremely low levels. There is some concern that irradiation of foods may result in induced radioactivity. Based on worst-case assumptions, the estimated induced radioactivity would be considerably below the level occurring naturally in food; irradiation in the commercially useful range is not expected to generate measurable additional radioactivity in foods.

3. Post-irradiation detection

Ideally, analytical methods to detect whether, and to what extent, foods have been irradiated should be simple, rapid, and reliable, use ordinary instruments and small samples, and be applicable to all food types. Realistically, such methods will not be available in the near future, and methods of analysis will almost certainly vary with food type and with the nature of the analyte.

The detection of chemical changes in food has been the basis of a number of analytical approaches. Much progress has been made over the past 10 years in the development of techniques to detect and measure changes in proteins, lipids, carbohydrates and other food components. Physical properties have also been investigated, including changes in electrical impedance, electric potential, and viscosity. Techniques using thermal analysis, near-infrared analysis, and electron spin resonance have had some success, and measurement of induced luminescence shows promise. Biological changes are also being studied as a means of detecting food irradiation.

Many of these approaches have been or are being tested in international collaborative studies. While no truly specific methods of detecting food treated by irradiation exist as yet, future work, especially that involving DNA, may well lead to such methods applicable to nearly all food types. Several methods tested in collaborative trials have been found to be suitable for a number of foods.

4. Toxicology

Very large numbers of animal studies have been carried out over the past few decades, but no evidence has been found of adverse effects resulting from the consumption of irradiated food. Where differences have been noted between control and test animals, no consistent patterns have been observed in type of abnormality, type of food, amount consumed, duration of study and radiation dose.

Hundreds of studies covering all aspects of toxicology, including chronic and subchronic effects, reproduction, teratology, and mutagenesis, have been evaluated. Despite some deficiencies in a number of the studies reviewed, the consistency with which the studies report the absence of adverse toxicological effects following consumption of irradiated food is remarkable.

The studies carried out by Raltech, a well known testing laboratory in the USA, in which 134 tonnes of irradiated chicken meat were fed to laboratory animals, are among the most comprehensive ever conducted, and included chronic studies in two species, teratology studies in four species, a dominant lethal study, a sex-linked recessive test, and an Ames mutagenicity test. The results showed a general lack of effects associated with the treatment, providing further evidence that the consumption of irradiated food does not pose a hazard.

A large number of animal feeding studies have been carried out by the International Project in the Field of Food Irradiation (IFIP). The project was in existence from 1970 to 1982 and produced over 70 reports describing the feeding studies undertaken, none of which demonstrated any adverse effects of irradiation.

In 1987, a collection of toxicity studies was submitted to the FDA in support of a petition proposing the use of irradiation of poultry products to extend shelf-life and reduce the risk posed by *Salmonella*. The submission included three feeding studies carried out in the Netherlands, at the Central Institute for Nutrition and Food Research. The investigations included a multigeneration study in rats, a chronic study in rats, and a 1-year toxicity study in dogs. No treatment-related adverse effects were noted.

Considerable attention has been given to several studies reporting the induction of polyploidy following the consumption of irradiated wheat by mammalian species or malnourished children. The results of these studies were found, after careful examination, not to be materially different from those of more extensive and statistically valid studies showing no effect of consumption of irradiated wheat on polyploidy.

Overall, no adverse effects of feeding irradiated foods to animals have been observed, and it is concluded that the irradiation of foods in accordance with established good manufacturing practices raises no unresolved questions of safety.

5. Microbiology

Ionizing radiation produces chemical changes that may kill or inactivate microorganisms. Most applications are at dose levels insufficient to kill all the microorganisms present, but sufficient to cause significant reductions in their number and variety. Doses between 2 and 7 kGy result in extensive destruction of common foodborne microorganisms, virtually eliminating organisms such as *Salmonella*. The shelf-life of foods can thereby be extended, and the threat of illness from pathogenic organisms eliminated or greatly reduced.

On the other hand, doses up to 50 kGy are necessary to eliminate highly resistant spores of organisms such as *Clostridium botulinum*. Comprehensive studies on chicken and fish inoculated at extremely high levels have shown that enough spoilage organisms remain after irradiation to produce the tell-tale signs of decomposition if the food is subsequently stored improperly. Although differential growth is possible, this does not represent a hazard unique to irradiation, nor one that cannot be effectively managed by using microbiological and other conventional techniques.

Concern that irradiation will result in increased induction of mutants that may possess increased pathogenicity, virulence, or radiation resistance has been expressed, but there is no scientific evidence that such transformations take place. Irradiation is by no means unique in its potential to increase the rate of mutation. Conventional processing techniques may also increase mutation rates, yet no evidence has been found to show that they have increased the pathogenicity or virulence of pathogenic organisms.

Finally, there has been concern over possible increased production of aflatoxin following irradiation. The evidence is mixed, but the overall scientific information indicates that irradiated food stored under typical conditions does not generate elevated aflatoxin levels.

In summary, there is no reason to suppose that irradiated food need be subjected to controls different from those regularly applied to food processed by conventional means.

6. Nutrition

Among the most important issues to be considered in assessing the acceptability of irradiated foods is whether such foods are nutritionally equivalent to those processed by traditional means. Food irradiation can cause changes in both macro- and micronutrients, but these changes are small. Irradiation is not alone in its ability to produce nutritional changes. Many food processes, notably cooking and heating in general, also cause nutrient loss, often to a greater extent than irradiation. The energy value of foods depends on the proteins, carbohydrates, and fats in them. At irradiation doses up to 10 kGy, no significant destruction of these macronutrients has been observed. While chemical analyses do show effects with doses up to and including sterilizing doses (50 kGy), they are small and nonspecific.

The view that irradiated foods are generally nutritionally equivalent to nonirradiated foods subjected to normal processing is supported by many animal studies, including some in which the protein efficiency ratio for many irradiated high-protein foods was measured. Proteins are of special concern, as they provide essential amino acids needed by the body to build its own protein. No significant effects on essential amino acids have been observed in beef, fish, or many other foodstuffs, in some cases at sterilizing doses.

The effect of irradiation on vitamins varies depending on the food type, the vitamin in question, and the process and storage conditions. Some vitamins are fairly insensitive to irradiation; others are more easily destroyed. The importance of a vitamin loss in any particular food depends on the contribution of that food to the total diet. For example, loss of vitamins from spices would not be a cause for concern, but loss of thiamine (vitamin B_1) from pork could be detrimental to populations where pork is an important component of the diet.

There is no loss of minerals and trace elements as these nutrients are unaffected by irradiation.

Irradiation temperature, exposure to air, and storage conditions may all affect nutrient content. In many cases, low-temperature irradiation in the absence of oxygen helps to reduce any losses of vitamins in foods, and storage of irradiated foods in sealed packages at low temperature also helps to prevent future decomposition.

7. Conclusions

A review of the available scientific literature indicates that food irradiation is a thoroughly tested food technology. Safety studies have so far shown no deleterious effects. Irradiation will help to ensure a safer and more plentiful food supply by extending shelf-life and by inactivating pests and pathogens. As long as requirements for good manufacturing practice are implemented, food irradiation is safe and effective. Possible risks resulting from disregard of good manufacturing practice are not basically different from those resulting from abuses of other processing methods, such as canning, freezing and pasteurization.

1.
Introduction

All governments bear direct or indirect responsibility for ensuring sufficient supplies of safe, nutritious, and acceptable food to meet the needs of their people. Such supplies should be of high quality and comprise a wide variety of foodstuffs.

Achieving the objective of sustaining or expanding high-quality food supplies is made difficult by agroclimatic conditions, the lack of technology, the seasonality of production, and the perishable nature of many crops. All countries depend to some extent on food processing and preservation technology. The need for treatment and preservation of food is currently being met through a variety of processes, some of which, such as drying and salting, are of considerable antiquity, while others, such as fumigation, canning and pasteurization, are of more recent origin.

Treatment by ionizing radiation is now beginning to be used to supplement existing technologies for certain applications. One such application, which has potential public health benefits, is the reduction of the numbers of pathogenic microorganisms in solid foods. Irradiation, as a process used to meet quarantine requirements, also has great promise as an alternative both to other physical methods and to fumigation.

Before this new food processing technology could be introduced, clear evidence and assurance had to be obtained that not only would it produce the desired results but also that it would not have any unacceptable toxicological, nutritional, and microbiological effects. The task of gathering this information at the international level was coordinated by the International Project in the Field of Food Irradiation (IFIP), which began in 1970. The data generated by this project and obtained from other sources were reviewed at a series of international meetings organized by the World Health Organization (WHO), often jointly with the Food and Agriculture Organization of the United Nations (FAO) and the International Atomic Energy Agency (IAEA). In 1980, these international deliberations culminated in the convening at WHO headquarters in Geneva of a Joint FAO/IAEA/WHO Expert Committee on the Wholesomeness of Irradiated Food.

In their landmark report (WHO, 1981), the Committee concluded that the "irradiation of any food commodity up to an overall average dose of 10 kGy presents no toxicological hazard; hence, toxicological testing of foods so treated is no longer required." It also found that irradiation up to 10 kGy "introduces no special nutritional or microbiological problems". The conclusions of the Expert Committee, then, clearly established the wholesomeness of irradiated food up to this maximum absorbed dose of 10 kGy.

Subsequently, a number of national authorities convened their own expert committees to review and evaluate the data. Reviews were conducted, for example, in Denmark, France, the United Kingdom and the United States of America, and by the Scientific Committee for Food of the European Economic Community. All these reviews arrived at the same conclusion as was reached by WHO, FAO and IAEA in 1980.

On the basis of the report of the Joint FAO/IAEA/WHO Expert Committee on the Wholesomeness of Irradiated Food, as well as of information available from national expert committees and other relevant information, the Joint FAO/WHO Codex Alimentarius Commission, in consultation with its member countries, reviewed the use of irradiation as a food technology and at its fifteenth session in 1983 adopted the Codex General Standard for Irradiated Foods and the Recommended International Code of Practice for the Operation of Radiation Facilities used for the Treatment of Food (FAO, 1984). With the endorsement of the Commission, FAO and WHO expressed the hope that countries would begin in earnest to apply food irradiation for the full benefit of their people, regardless of the stage of development reached.

There has been considerable opposition on the part of several consumer organizations to the introduction of this technology. On a number of occasions, WHO and other international organizations have responded to the concerns expressed (IAEA, 1989; WHO, 1988, 1989). There have been many examples in the past where public health advice on new technologies has not been immediately accepted, pasteurization of milk being a good case in point. When it was introduced about 100 years ago in North America, Europe, and other parts of the world, many milk consumers, as well as some scientists, voiced objections based on perceived hygienic, nutritional and economic concerns. Today, pasteurization of milk is universally accepted as an essential public health technology that enjoys the confidence and support of the public.

Whereas pasteurization was introduced mainly to interrupt the transmission of bovine tuberculosis and brucellosis, the most important public health application of food irradiation is to destroy or reduce the ubiquitous and largely unavoidable pathogens that contaminate raw foods, especially those of animal origin. In view of the enormous health and economic consequences of foodborne diseases, decontamination of certain foods by irradiation should be seriously considered.

References

FAO (1984) *Codex General Standard for Irradiated Foods and Recommended International Code of Practice for the Operation of Radiation Facilities Used for the Treatment of Food*. Rome, Food and Agriculture Organization of the United Nations.

IAEA (1989) *Acceptance, control of, and trade in irradiated food*. Vienna, International Atomic Energy Agency.

WHO (1981) *Wholesomeness of irradiated food: report of a joint FAO/IAEA/WHO Expert Committee*. Geneva, World Health Organization (WHO Technical Report Series, No. 659).

WHO (1988) *Food irradiation. A technique for preserving and improving the safety of food*. Geneva, World Health Organization.

WHO (1989) *Consumer concerns about the safety of food—the WHO reply to questions raised by the International Organization of Consumers Unions (IOCU)*. Geneva, World Health Organization (unpublished document WHO/EHE/FOS/89.1; available on request from Food Safety, World Health Organization, 1211 Geneva 27, Switzerland).

2.
Food irradiation

2.1 History of food preservation

On a global scale, between a quarter and a half of the world's food supply is lost post-harvest as a result of spoilage, insect infestation, and bacterial and fungal attack (WHO, 1988). However, the loss of edible food is only part of a larger problem. In 1983, a Joint FAO/WHO Expert Committee on Food Safety concluded that foodborne disease, while not well documented, was one of the most widespread threats to human health and an important cause of reduced productivity (WHO, 1984). It is estimated that foodborne diarrhoeal diseases account for up to 70% of the 3.2 million deaths in children under the age of five, worldwide.

Food loss resulting from inadequate storage conditions is not a new problem and devising ways to prevent it has been a major concern throughout history. There is archaeological evidence that the drying of strips of meat and split fish was practised in early civilizations (Hugo, 1991). With the domestication of animals and the development of agricultural skills, food preservation techniques became more sophisticated and included fermentation, smoking, drying, salting, freezing and cooking.

Delicacies such as bananas and pineapples became available in 16th century England, not so much because food preservation techniques had progressed but because post-harvest delivery time had been shortened (Stewart & Amerine, 1973). In 1809, the French Government offered a prize for a method of preserving food. Nicholas Appert won the prize a year later with his method of sealing vegetables and fruit in glass jars and then heating the jars (Hugo, 1991). During the American Civil War (circa 1860), the canning industry greatly expanded and canned goods became a general item of issue, especially in the Northern army (Stewart & Amerine, 1973). The development of artificial refrigeration for ships and railcars had a profound effect on the movement of bulk quantities of produce and meat (Stewart & Amerine, 1973).

An important advance in food preservation, which had a significant impact on public health, was the introduction of pasteurization at the turn of the century. The process had been developed in France in the 1860s by Dr Louis Pasteur to improve the keeping quality of wine and beer, and a decade later was applied to milk by Professor N. J. Fjord in Denmark. In spite of the public health benefits of pasteurization, especially the dramatic reduction in infant mortality, controversy delayed its widespread introduction. One of the objections raised at that time was that pasteurization would be used to hide poor-quality and improperly handled milk. In fact, the New York City Board of Health in 1906 prohibited secret pasteurization for this reason. Fortunately, following studies conducted by the US Public Health Service, pasteurization gradually became accepted as an important public health measure and, in 1909, the first compulsory pasteurization law in the United States was adopted by the city of Chicago. Today, pasteurization of milk and other liquid foods is unquestioned as an essential process for ensuring the safety of these products while at the same time extending their shelf-lives.

Just as the American Civil War had stimulated technological advances in the canning industry, so the Second World War stimulated advances in dehydration technology. At the end of the war, dehydrated milk, eggs, onions, carrots, cabbage, potatoes and other foods of satisfactory quality were being produced in large quantities.

Although irradiation as a method of food preservation had been explored as early as 1905 and was proposed by the US Department of Agriculture in 1916 as a method of ridding cigars of the destructive tobacco beetle, the technology for developing a consistent, reliable and economic source of radiation was not then available. Finally, after the Second World War, the US Atomic Energy Commission, exploring constructive uses of irradiation, was instrumental in installing food irradiators at several universities. In addition, an irradiator was installed in the National Marine Fisheries Service in 1964, followed by another in 1965 at the US Department of Agriculture Entomological Research Center for use with grain products (Diehl, 1990).

Probably the greatest stimulus to the use of irradiation for food preservation in the United States was provided by the United States Army, which started work as early as 1953, and in 1960 decided to concentrate on radiation as a method of meat sterilization in place of canning or freezing (Diehl, 1990).

Work was not confined to the United States, however. As early as 1950, work had begun at the Low Temperature Research Station at Cambridge, England, and in the mid-to-late 1950s programmes were under way in Belgium, Canada, France, the Federal Republic of Germany, the Netherlands, Poland and the Soviet Union.

2.2 Radiation sources

Food irradiation calls for the carefully controlled exposure of food materials under specific environmental conditions to a source of ionizing radiation of known energy. The exposure must be adequate to produce the desired result, but at the same time degradation of the food product must be avoided.

Guidelines exist in many countries defining the minimum and maximum exposures for various commodities.

To produce the predictable, precise amount of ionizing energy necessary to achieve an adequate exposure, four sources of radiation are of potential interest, namely cobalt-60, caesium-137, and electron beam and X-ray generators. Of these, only cobalt-60 and electron beam generators have achieved major importance. Each of the sources has specific advantages and disadvantages.

To obtain cobalt-60, highly refined cobalt-59 pellets are converted into a radioactive gamma source in a nuclear reactor via neutron activation. The pellets are placed in a stainless steel capsule in the form of a "pin" or "pencil" to minimize self-absorption and heat build-up. With this configuration, about 95% of the emitted energy is available for use. The specific radioactive strength of emission of each pencil is determined and the pencils are then placed in a holder in an arrangement of known total strength of emission.

The advantages of cobalt-60 as a source are: (1) high penetration and good dose uniformity, allowing treatment of products of variable size, shape and density; (2) a long history of satisfactory use in similar applications; (3) ready availability of several sources of this material and (4) low environmental risk. Disadvantages include: (1) a half-life of 5.3 years, so that 12% of the source must be replaced annually to maintain the original strength; and (2) a rather slow food processing rate compared with electron beam irradiation (Jarrett, 1982). Despite these drawbacks, cobalt-60 is the radiation source of choice.

Caesium-137 is also a gamma-ray emitter. It is produced as a result of uranium fission and may be reclaimed as a by-product of nuclear fuel reprocessing. Construction of reprocessing plants on a large scale was planned in several countries in the 1960s and 1970s, and the use of caesium-137 as a source of gamma radiation was promulgated at that time. However, for a number of reasons, the reprocessing plants were not built and caesium-137 is therefore not available in sufficiently large quantities to play a role in commercial food irradiation. There is no indication that this situation will change in the foreseeable future, and cobalt-60 is therefore the only gamma source of practical interest.

When not in use, gamma sources are generally stored under water, which provides efficient shielding. The sources are removed from the pool and taken into a room shielded with concrete, where they are allowed to irradiate the target food, which is brought in on a conveyor. At the end of the exposure period, the source is simply lowered into the pool by a mechanical device.

Neither cobalt-60 nor caesium-137 will contribute to long-term radioactive waste since cobalt-60 decays to form nonradioactive nickel and caesium-137 decays to give nonradioactive barium.

In contrast to the gamma-emitting isotope sources, the radiation from electron beam and X-ray machines is produced electrically, resulting in considerable on-site power consumption. The practical usefulness of all electron accelerators depends on the energy of the ionizing radiation and, when electrons are used directly, the short depth of penetration limits their use in food applications. Electron linear accelerators (linacs) can be designed to produce electron energies sufficient to reach the maximum of 10 MeV allowed for food irradiation (Ramler, 1982; FAO, 1984).

Even with the higher-energy linacs, the relatively shallow depth of penetration of the electron beams prevents their use in the irradiation of animal carcasses or other thick materials. Conversion of these electron beams into X-rays overcomes the penetration problem. Since the X-rays are at least as penetrating as the gamma rays of cobalt-60, uniform penetration of foods can also be achieved.

The major advantage of the accelerator and X-ray generator as compared with the gamma irradiators is that they can simply be turned off when not in use. Additional advantages include the following: (1) the source does not need to be replenished; (2) they are readily available; (3) they have an established history of use; and (4) they have a high throughput rate. Disadvantages include: (1) the complexity of the machine and the consequent need for regular maintenance; and (2) the large requirements for power and cooling. As mentioned earlier, the main difference between the electrons produced by an accelerator and X-rays is that the penetration of the latter is greater.

The process of food irradiation when an accelerator producing electrons or X-rays is used differs little from that when sources of gamma rays are employed. The food target is passed on a conveyor through a labyrinth of shielding to the irradiator, where it is irradiated at the appropriate exposure level. During irradiation with either radioisotopes or machine sources, dosimeters are placed at strategic positions in the food container to measure the absorbed dose throughout the food.

Short-lived radioactive isotopes may be formed in food irradiated with electrons or X-rays of sufficiently high energy (X-rays are more efficient in inducing radioactivity than electrons of the same energy). These isotopes can be produced at energies as low as 14 MeV with X-rays and 20 MeV with electrons. As a precaution, a maximum energy level of 10 MeV for electrons and 5 MeV for gamma rays and X-rays was recommended by the Joint FAO/IAEA/WHO Expert Committee on the Wholesomeness of Irradiated Food (WHO, 1981) and endorsed by the Codex Alimentarius Commission (FAO, 1984).

2.3 Mechanism of food irradiation

Radiation destroys microbial contaminants, including spoilage organisms, by the partial or total inactivation of the genetic material of the living cells in food, either by its direct effects on DNA or through the production of radicals and ions that attack DNA.

It is important to remember that food irradiation under the recommended conditions does not involve the atomic nucleus itself, but rather the electron cloud surrounding the nucleus, which initiates a purely chemical reaction. The consequent effects on biological materials are the sum of the direct or primary, and the indirect or secondary effects (Moseley, 1989).

The primary effect is produced by energetic electrons (emanating from the source or produced through Compton scattering) and may result in one or more of three outcomes: (1) ionization (removal of an electron); (2) dissociation (loss of a hydrogen atom); or (3) excitation (raising of the molecule to a higher energy level). As a result of the highly reactive free radicals produced, a number of secondary reactions may occur, e.g. recombination, dimerization or electron capture, involving other molecules present in the complex mixture constituting the food (see Chapter 4). Disproportionation may also occur, producing a substance which may not have been present originally.

The breaking of chemical bonds by radiation is called radiolysis. It produces unstable reactive products that are subsequently converted to stable end-products. The tendency is for there to be a linear relationship between the radiation dose and the amount of radiolytic products generated, i.e. a doubling of the radiation dose will double the amount of such products formed. Virtually all radiolytic products have been found to be the same as thermolytic and photolytic products produced by heating and exposure to light, respectively (Diehl, 1990).

As discussed in Chapter 4, factors other than dose strongly influence the nature and amount of radiolytic products formed. The presence of water or oxygen and the relative amounts thereof can have a profound influence on the radiolytic process.

The temperature and the physical state of the food can also affect the outcome of the process. Freezing, for example, has a protective effect during irradiation by preventing the products of water radiolysis from reacting with the substrate. On warming, these products (hydroxyl radicals) tend to react preferentially with each other rather than with the substrate, so that damage to the latter is often less when it is irradiated in the frozen state. Anaerobic conditions also influence the nature of the radiolytic products, since the presence of oxygen during irradiation can generate highly reactive superoxide radicals, peroxy radicals and hydrogen peroxide.

Macronutrients, in the presence of water, interact primarily with hydroxyl radicals which, in turn, react predominantly with hydrogen bonded to carbon atoms (hydrogen abstraction). The resulting free radicals may initiate a number of reactions (see Chapter 4). The overall effect is a series of hydrolyses and oxidative degradations. Some of the radiolytic products formed from carbohydrates consist of increased amounts of sugar acids and ketones, oligosaccharides yielding monosaccharides and polysaccharides yielding smaller units (CAST, 1986). Proteins undergo abstraction of hydrogen by both hydroxyl radicals and hydrogen radicals, and reductive deamination (in the presence of oxygen, oxidative deamination). The resulting radicals undergo further reactions.

In contrast to protein and carbohydrates, where radiolytic activity is mainly via water and therefore indirect, the primary effect in fats is direct, cation radicals or excited molecules being formed (see Chapter 4). Other reactions will involve excited triglycerides, and the presence of double bonds will result in the generation of additional products. The main reactions therefore involve oxidation, polymerization, decarboxylation and dehydration (CAST, 1986). These changes affect less than 0.2% of the total lipids (at absorbed doses up to 50 kGy[1]) and do not change the nutritional value of the food (CAST, 1986). The presence of proteins or carbohydrates will reduce the amount of radiolytic products generated from fats (see Chapter 4 on chemistry and Chapter 5 on post-irradiation detection methods).

Micronutrients may also be affected by food irradiation, and this is discussed in Chapter 8.

Initial products associated with radiolysis, e.g. superoxide radicals, hydrogen peroxide, hydroperoxides and others, are chemically very reactive and tend to disappear quickly, especially in an aqueous medium. Even with dried foods, such as spices, radicals will react quickly to form stable radiolytic products when they are added to water-containing foods (Thayer, 1990).

2.4 Activity in biological systems

For a living biological system, chromosomal DNA is the most critical target of irradiation, although other cellular components may also be affected. The direct effect of irradiation on nucleic acid molecules is either ionization or excitation. Indirect effects on DNA include excitation of water molecules which then diffuse in the medium and may make contact with the chromosomal material. An exposure of 0.1 kGy results in 2.8% of the DNA being damaged whereas 0.14% of enzymes and 0.005% of amino acids are altered with the same dose (Diehl, 1990).

The Brynjolfsson formula[2] estimates the probability that a molecule will change at a given dose of irradiation (Brynjolfsson, 1981). At 10 kGy, 72 of every million water molecules at most will be affected, but DNA, with its high relative molecular mass of 10^9, will undergo 4000 changes per molecule. Most of these changes are single-strand breaks, and are not lethal to an organism. The G value for double-strand breaks, which are usually lethal, is

---

[1] The gray (Gy) is the unit of absorbed dose of ionizing energy, and is equivalent to 1 joule/kg. The gray replaces the rad (radiation absorbed dose) as the unit of absorbed dose. One gray is equivalent to 100 rads.
[2] $X = 10^{-7} \times G \times M \times D$
where X = the average no. of changes per molecule on irradiation; G = the number of changes per 100 eV of absorbed energy ($G \leq 4$ in aqueous systems); M = relative molecular mass; and D = dose in kGy.

about 0.07, so that DNA will undergo 70 double-strand breaks per molecule — lethal for living organisms, but of no consequence for food.

One goal of food irradiation is to reduce the contaminant microbial population. The mean lethal dose (MLD) is defined as the dose required to kill 63% of a population (D_{37}). However, D_{10}, the dose required to kill 90% of the population, is more commonly used. D_{10} depends on a variety of factors including the food to be irradiated, the temperature, the presence of oxygen, and the water content. All these factors, including post-irradiation storage conditions (for nonsterilizing doses), determine the ultimate fitness of the food for human consumption.

The radiation sensitivity of yeasts and moulds is not measured in terms of D_{10}, but of the dose required to reach a specific end-point. For example, the lowest dose that ensures that a specific number of spores in the inoculum do not survive is the inactivation dose. Other measures include post-irradiation colony size for a specific number of spores following a specified number of days of growth, and the dose of radiation required to inhibit a specific function, such as carbon dioxide production by fermentation yeasts. As with bacteria, post-irradiation environmental conditions (e.g. temperature) can influence survival.

Though radiation may inactivate organisms or even sterilize food, many of their products, whether mycotoxins or bacterial toxins, are radiation-resistant and cannot be inactivated at practical dose levels, so that toxin-contaminated food cannot be detoxified through irradiation. In this regard, irradiation does not differ from conventional methods of pasteurization or sterilization by heat, which also do not destroy most microbial toxins.

Viruses representing significant health hazards in food include those causing hepatitis and poliomyelitis. They can also be inactivated by irradiation, the rate of inactivation being an exponential function of dose. As in the case of bacteria, yeasts or moulds, the inactivation dose for a type of virus will depend on the initial level of contamination. Viruses tend to be relatively resistant to radiation and a dose of 10 kGy may eliminate only 99% of those present. They are not inactivated by freezing, but are sensitive to heat. A combination of heat treatment and irradiation may therefore be the most useful procedure for inactivating microbial pathogens, including viruses. For hepatitis A virus in clams and oysters, a D_{10} of 2 kGy has been recorded (Mallet et al., 1991).

It has been suggested that the use of irradiation may result in the production of a "superbug" (bacterium or virus) that would be radiation-resistant (Murray, 1990). Added to this concern is the idea that resistance to radiation would be associated with increased virulence. While it is true that the use of radiation has led to the discovery of radiation-resistant organisms such as *Moraxella acinetobacter* and *Deinococcus* (formerly *Micrococcus*) *radiodurans* (CAST, 1986), there is no record of the formation of a truly superior species either through selection or mutation. In its response to this concern, the FDA (Food and Drug Administration, 1986) commented that:

> Mutants produced during irradiation of food are essentially the same as those that occur naturally. The only real difference is in the rate at which mutations occur. Nor is there any reason to expect that the resulting mutants would be different or more virulent than those created by nature.

On the whole, most of the mutations induced by irradiation are not advantageous to the bacterial species, such mutants tending not to survive and to be less robust than previous generations; they are usually poor competitors with the nonmutated strains (Australian House of Representatives, 1988; CAST, 1989).

A number of protozoa and parasitic helminths are pathogenic to humans; most can be killed or rendered noninfectious at doses under 1.0 kGy.

The radiation dose required to kill an insect pest will depend on the type of insect and the specific stage in the life cycle. For instance, radiation sensitivity is greatest in the insect during the egg stage and lowest in the adult. Although up to 3 kGy are required to kill all individuals at all stages, lower doses may inhibit continued maturation or cause sterilization. There are species differences among insects and other arthropod pests in susceptibility to radiation, moths being more resistant than mites, and beetles most sensitive. In general, 0.5 kGy will control most resistant beetles and immature moths, and the offspring of the moths will be sterile. Insects are known for their ability to develop resistance to pesticides but this has not been found for radiation (Tilton & Brower, 1987). Tilton & Burditt (1983) found that insect survivors of radiation exhibited reduced fitness and shorter life spans.

2.5 Previous reviews

Numerous international and national meetings, conferences and workshops have addressed the topic of food irradiation over the past 30 years. Among these are several activities sponsored by specialized agencies of the United Nations, including joint activities of WHO, FAO and IAEA; these are listed below in chronological order:

1. A joint FAO/WHO/IAEA meeting on the wholesomeness of irradiated foods—with exclusive reference to the evaluation of nutritional adequacy and safety for consumption, Brussels, October 1961 (FAO, 1962).
2. A joint FAO/IAEA/WHO Expert Committee meeting on the technical basis for legislation on irradiated food, Rome, April 1964 (WHO, 1966).

3. A joint FAO/IAEA/WHO Expert Committee meeting on the wholesomeness of irradiated food with special reference to wheat, potatoes and onions, Geneva, April 1969 (WHO, 1970).
4. A joint FAO/IAEA/WHO Expert Committee meeting on the wholesomeness of irradiated food, Geneva, August/September 1976 (WHO, 1977).
5. A joint FAO/IAEA/WHO Expert Committee meeting on the wholesomeness of irradiated food, Geneva, 27 October–3 November 1980. This meeting was a major turning point in the scientific evaluation of the safety of irradiated foods. Two conclusions are of major importance in the context of safety and nutritional quality: (1) "irradiation of any food commodity up to an overall average dose of 10 kGy presents no toxicological hazard; hence, toxicological testing of foods so treated is no longer required"; and (2) "irradiation of food up to an overall average dose of 10 kGy introduces no special nutritional or microbiological problems" (WHO, 1981).
6. A meeting of the Board of the International Committee on Food Microbiology and Hygiene (ICFMH), with the participation of WHO, FAO and IAEA, on the microbiological safety of irradiated foods, Copenhagen, 1982 (FAO, 1983).
7. Adoption of the Codex General Standard for Irradiated Foods and the Recommended International Code of Practice for the Operation of Radiation Facilities Used for the Treatment of Food by the Joint WHO/FAO Codex Alimentarius Commission, in 1983. These established the basic principles for the irradiation of foods on a worldwide basis (FAO, 1984).
8. Publication of the book *Food irradiation. A technique for preserving and improving the safety of food* (WHO, 1988).
9. International Conference on the Acceptance, Control of, and Trade in Irradiated Food, Geneva, 1988. This conference was organized jointly by FAO, WHO, IAEA and the International Trade Centre, and was attended by representatives of governments and governmental and nongovernmental organizations. The Conference adopted, by consensus, an International Document on Food Irradiation which recommended the following:

   (a) Consideration should be given to the application of food irradiation technology for public health benefits, especially for products where this process would seem advantageous.
   (b) Consideration should be given to the application of food irradiation technology where it can, in appropriate cases, reduce postharvest losses of food and serve as a quarantine treatment.
   (c) Governments should ensure that, as a prerequisite to any processing of food by irradiation or sale of irradiated food, regulatory

procedures for control are introduced. The key principles on which such procedures should be based are the registration/licensing, regulation and inspection of food irradiation facilities, the documentation and labelling of irradiated food, the training of control officials, and the employment of good manufacturing practices.

(d) Regulatory procedures for the control of the food irradiation process should be consistent with the internationally agreed principles embodied in the Codex General Standard for Irradiated Foods and associated Code of Practice. The radiation doses administered should be measured by methods meeting national or international standards so as to provide a means of independent verification.

(e) Governments should encourage research on methods of detection of irradiated food so that administrative control of such food once it leaves the facility can be supplemented by an additional means of enforcement, thus facilitating international trade and strengthening consumer confidence in the overall system.

(f) The labelling of irradiated food for international trade should be in line with the provisions adopted by the Codex Alimentarius Commission.

(g) Governments should ensure that all phases of the planning and operation of food irradiation facilities are subject to a regulatory structure consistent with relevant internationally accepted standards for human health, safety and environmental protection.

(h) Governments, especially those that plan to authorize food irradiation, should be encouraged to provide clear and adequate information about the process to the public. The active participation of all interested parties, including consumers, should be encouraged.

The document reconfirmed the conclusions of the 1980 meeting of the Joint Expert Committee and reaffirmed the validity of the Codex Standard described above. The full proceedings of this conference were published in 1989 (IAEA, 1989).

References

Australian House of Representatives (Standing Committee on Environment, Recreation and the Arts) (1988) *Use of ionising radiation.* Canberra, Australian Government Publishing Service.

Brynjolfsson A (1981) Chemiclearance of food irradiation: its scientific basis. In: *Combination processes in food irradiation. Proceedings of a symposium held in Colombo, November 1980.* Vienna, International Atomic Energy Agency, pp. 367–374.

CAST (1986) *Ionizing energy in food processing and pest control. I. Wholesomeness of food treated with ionizing energy*. Ames, IA, Council for Agricultural Science and Technology (Task Force Report No. 109).

CAST (1989) *Ionizing energy in food processing and pest control. II. Applications*. Ames, IA, Council for Agricultural Science and Technology (Task Force Report No. 115).

Diehl JF (1990) *The safety of irradiated food*. New York and Basel, Marcel Dekker.

FAO (1962) *Report of the FAO/WHO/IAEA Meeting on the Wholesomeness of Irradiated Foods, Brussels, 23–30 October 1961*. Rome, Food and Agriculture Organization of the United Nations.

FAO (1983) *The microbiological safety of irradiated food*. Rome, Food and Agriculture Organization of the United Nations (unpublished document of the Codex Alimentarius Commission No. CX/FH 83/9).

FAO (1984) *Codex General Standard for Irradiated Foods and Recommended International Code of Practice for the Operation of Radiation Facilities Used for the Treatment of Food*. Rome, Food and Agriculture Organization of the United Nations (CAC/Vol XV-Ed. 1).

Food and Drug Administration (1986) Irradiation in the production, processing and handling of food, *Federal register*, **51**:13376.

Hugo WB (1991) A brief history of heat and chemical preservation and disinfection. *Journal of applied bacteriology*, **71**:9–18.

IAEA (1989) *Acceptance, control of, and trade in irradiated food*. Vienna, International Atomic Energy Agency.

Jarrett RD Sr (1982) Isotope (gamma) radiation sources. In: Josephson ES, Peterson MS, eds. *Preservation of food by ionizing radiation*, Vol 1, Boca Raton, FL, CRC Press, pp. 137–163.

Mallet JC et al. (1991) Potential of irradiation technology for improved shellfish sanitation. *Journal of food safety*, **11**:231–245.

Moseley BEB (1989) Ionizing radiation: action and repair. In: Gould GW, ed., *Mechanisms of action of food preservation procedures*. New York, Elsevier Applied Science, pp. 43–70.

Murray DR (1990) *Biology of food irradiation*. New York, Wiley.

Ramler WJ (1982) Machine sources. In: Josephson ES, Peterson MS, eds. *Preservation of food by ionizing radiation*, Vol. 1, Boca Raton, FL, CRC Press, pp. 165–187.

Stewart GF, Amerine MA (1973) Evolution of food processing. In: *Introduction to food science and technology*. New York, Academic Press, pp. 1–26.

Thayer DW (1990) Food irradiation: benefits and concerns. *Journal of food quality*, **13**:147–169.

Tilton EW, Brower JH (1987) Ionizing radiation for insect control in grain and grain products. *Cereal foods world*, **32**:330–335.

Tilton EW, Burditt AK Jr (1983) Insect disinfestation of grain and fruit. In: Josephson ES, Peterson MS, eds. *Preservation of food by ionizing radiation*, Vol. 3. Boca Raton, FL, CRC Press, pp. 215–229.

WHO (1966) *The technical basis for legislation on irradiated food: report of a Joint FAO/IAEA/WHO Expert Committee*. Geneva, World Health Organization (WHO Technical Report Series, No. 316).

WHO (1970) *Wholesomeness of irradiated food with special reference to wheat, potatoes and onions: report of a Joint FAO/IAEA/WHO Expert Committee*. Geneva, World Health Organization (WHO Technical Report Series, No. 451).

WHO (1977) *Wholesomeness of irradiated food: report of a Joint FAO/IAEA/WHO Expert Committee*. Geneva, World Health Organization (WHO Technical Report Series, No. 604).

WHO (1981) *Wholesomeness of irradiated food: report of a Joint FAO/IAEA/WHO Expert Committee*. Geneva, World Health Organization (WHO Technical Report Series, No. 659).

WHO (1984) *The role of food safety in health and development: report of a Joint FAO/WHO Expert Committee on Food Safety*. Geneva, World Health Organization (WHO Technical Report Series, No. 705).

WHO (1988) *Food irradiation. A technique for preserving and improving the safety of food*. Geneva, World Health Organization.

3.
Applications

3.1 Introduction

Treatment of food with ionizing radiation can produce a wide variety of beneficial effects, including: the extension of shelf-life; the destruction or inactivation of insects, parasites, pathogenic bacteria, moulds, and yeasts; the delay of ripening of fruits and vegetables; and the inhibition of post-harvest sprouting of tuber and bulb crops. Many of these effects can be achieved with relatively low radiation exposures.

Exposure to ionizing radiation produces changes in some of the food molecules. As far as is known, the molecules formed are the same as those naturally present in foods or formed by conventional processing such as cooking. Before government authorities can approve food irradiation processes, however, they must be sure that irradiated foods are wholesome, i.e. that the procedure has not resulted in any significant nutritional deficiencies, no toxic or radioactive chemicals have been produced, and microorganisms and their toxins are not present at harmful levels.

Treatments aimed at the inactivation of microorganisms were previously considered to fall into two groups—radiation sterilization and radiation pasteurization. For several reasons, these terms were unsatisfactory and, in 1964, a group of experts (Goresline et al., 1964) suggested three new terms, as follows:

1. *Radappertization:* the treatment of food with a dose of ionizing energy sufficient to prevent spoilage or toxicity of microbial origin no matter how long or under what conditions the food is stored after treatment, provided it is not recontaminated. This is also called sterilization. The required dose is usually in the range 25–45 kGy.
2. *Radicidation:* the treatment of food with a dose of ionizing energy sufficient to reduce the number of viable, non-spore-forming, pathogenic bacteria to such a level that none is detectable in the treated food when it is examined by any recognized bacteriological testing method. Such treatment also inactivates foodborne parasites. The required dose is in the range 2–8 kGy. The term may also be applied to the destruction of parasites such as tapeworm and *Trichinella* in meat, in which case the required dose is in the range 0.1–1 kGy.
3. *Radurization:* the treatment of food with a dose of ionizing energy sufficient to enhance its keeping quality by causing a substantial

reduction in the numbers of viable spoilage microorganisms. The required dose is in the range 0.4–10 kGy.

These terms are not used consistently in the literature.

3.2 Functions

Depending on the type of food and the irradiation dose, ionizing energy can have a variety of useful functions, as summarized in Table 1.

Table 1. Functions of food irradiation

Function	Dose (kGy)	Products irradiated
Low-dose (up to 1 kGy)		
(a) Inhibition of sprouting	0.05–0.15	Potatoes, onions, garlic, root ginger, etc.
(b) Insect disinfestation and parasite disinfection	0.15–0.5	Cereals and pulses, fresh and dried fruits, dried fish and meat, fresh pork, etc.
(c) Delay of physiological processes (e.g. ripening)	0.5–1.0	Fresh fruits and vegetables
Medium-dose (1–10 kGy)		
(a) Extension of shelf-life	1.0–3.0	Fresh fish, strawberries, etc.
(b) Elimination of spoilage and pathogenic microorganisms	1.0–7.0	Fresh and frozen seafood, raw or frozen poultry and meat, etc.
(c) Improving technological properties of food	2.0–7.0	Grapes (increasing juice yield), dehydrated vegetables (reduced cooking time), etc.
High dose (10–50 kGy)[a]		
(a) Industrial sterilization (in combination with mild heat)	30–50	Meat, poultry, seafood, prepared foods, sterilized hospital diets
(b) Decontamination of certain food additives and ingredients	10–50	Spices, enzyme preparations, natural gum, etc.

[a] Only used for special purposes. The Joint FAO/WHO Codex Alimentarius Commission has not yet endorsed high-dose applications.
Source: WHO (1988).

3.3 Plant products

Irradiation of fresh plant products is generally limited to low-dose applications, since higher doses harm these foodstuffs. The effects can vary significantly, depending on the type and variety of commodity, the quality, the degree of maturity, contamination with microbes, and treatment after harvest. Desirable results at doses up to 1 kGy include inhibition or delay of sprouting in tuber, bulb, and root crops; delay of ripening of some fruits; and insect disinfestation (Clarke, 1971; Staden, 1973; Urbain, 1978, 1986; Kader, 1986). Doses in the 1–3 kGy range can delay spoilage of some commodities, while severe destructive effects are generally observed at doses above 3 kGy.

3.3.1 Fresh fruits and vegetables

Inhibition of growth

Sprouting of crops such as potato, sweet potato, yam, onion, garlic, and Jerusalem artichoke is inhibited by doses in the range 0.05–0.15 kGy (Matsuyama & Umeda, 1983). The lowest effective dose varies among commodities and also among varieties of each commodity. Undesirable effects such as darkening, reduced vitamin content, and greater rotting in storage may be produced by higher doses. For many of these crops, the desired inhibitory effects can also be obtained by chemical treatment, e.g. maleic hydrazide, propham, and chlorpropham are effective sprout inhibitors (Matsuyama & Umeda, 1983; Thomas, 1984a,b). These chemicals, however, leave residues considered by some to be harmful, and many countries have prohibited their use (Diehl, 1990).

In temperate zones, untreated potatoes may be stored without sprouting for several months after harvest provided a low temperature (5 °C) is maintained. Those intended to be used for making potato chips are stored at 9–10 °C because a lower temperature promotes the formation of reducing sugars, causing undesirable browning on frying. Sprouting may begin as early as January in the northern hemisphere for the chip potatoes unless the crop is treated with a chemical sprout inhibitor or by irradiation. Radiation doses of 0.04–0.15 kGy are needed, depending on the variety of potato, the intended use, and the time between harvest and irradiation (Matsuyama & Umeda, 1983; Thomas, 1984a). A dose of 0.15 kGy effectively controls sprouting by inhibiting cell division. Potatoes treated in this way may be kept for as long as a year in a cool place (15 °C) without significant loss of quality. Inhibition of sprouting is most effective when potatoes are irradiated soon after harvest, while the tubers are still dormant. Later, higher doses are needed to achieve the same degree of inhibition.

A dose of 0.1 kGy can inhibit sprout formation in sweet potatoes. Lu et al. (1986) reported that the taste of baked sweet potatoes was unaffected at this dosage. The shelf-life of commonly used varieties in China (Province of

Taiwan) exposed to 0.05 kGy was increased from 1 month (nonirradiated) to about 5 months at ambient temperatures.

A dose of 0.02–0.04 kGy produces sprout inhibition in onions. Best results are obtained when the crop is irradiated soon after harvest, maximum inhibition resulting on exposure to radiation within 2 weeks (Thomas, 1984b). Some browning of the inner buds of the bulb may occur on long-term storage, but this does not appear to affect marketability (Grünewald, 1978; Curzio & Croci, 1983). Refrigeration near 0 °C or treatment with maleic hydrazide are also effective.

Irradiation of shallots and garlic soon after harvest (during dormancy) requires doses of only 0.02–0.06 kGy for complete inhibition of sprouting (Thomas, 1984b). A study carried out in the Republic of Korea (Kwon et al., 1985) concluded that a dose of 0.075 kGy would effectively inhibit sprouting even if applied some time after harvest.

Yams are a staple food in many tropical regions. Since only one crop can be harvested each year, long-term storage is critically important. Both refrigeration and chemical treatment are ineffective and traditional means of storage result in losses of up to 100% after 5–6 months. Irradiation trials (Adesuyi & Mackenzie, 1973) with the most common African variety were highly successful. Doses of 0.075–0.125 kGy inhibited sprouting and reduced rotting and weight loss for a period of 5 months. After 5 months of storage at ambient temperature, the taste quality of the yams dosed at 0.15 kGy was judged "very good" by tasters.

Insect disinfestation

Chemical fumigation is the most common treatment for insect control in fresh fruits and vegetables. Pesticides such as ethylene dibromide (EDB), methyl bromide, phosphine, ethylene oxide, and hydrogen cyanide have been used successfully for this purpose. Use of EDB and ethylene oxide is no longer permitted in many countries. Cold treatments and heat treatments are currently used for the control of insect pests in selected fruits. Methods such as the use of modified atmospheres, fumigation with naturally occurring volatile chemicals, ultrasound, microwaves, and different treatment combinations have also been explored (Couey, 1983).

Fruit flies, the mango seed weevil, the navel orange worm, the potato tuber worm, the codling moth, spider mites, scale insects, and other important pests may be controlled effectively with doses of less than 1 kGy (IAEA, 1973; Burditt, 1982; Tilton & Burditt, 1983; Moy, 1985). Most insects are sterilized at doses of 0.05–0.75 kGy. The emergence of adult fruit flies is prevented by a dose of 0.15 kGy, which has been suggested as a quarantine measure for fresh fruits and vegetables.

Sensitivity to irradiation

At doses of 0.25 kGy or less, most fruits and vegetables suffer no discernible damage (CAST, 1989). Some commodities may be damaged by doses between 0.25 and 1 kGy. Lettuce, artichokes, and other non-fruit vegetables are usually more radiation-sensitive than certain fruits and fruit-vegetables (e.g. apples, tomatoes, melons).

Kader (1986) classified fruits and fruit-vegetables into four groups according to their sensitivity to irradiation as follows:

Slight: apple, cherry, date, guava, longan, mango, muskmelon, nectarine, papaya, peach, rambutan, raspberry, strawberry, tamarillo, tomato.
Variable: apricot, banana, cherimoya, fig, grapefruit, kumquat, lychee, loquat, orange, passion fruit, pear, pineapple, plum, tangelo, tangerine.
Serious: avocado, cucumber, grape, green bean, lemon, lime, olive, pepper, sapodilla, soursop, summer squash.
No data: kiwi fruit, pomegranate.

Delay of ripening and senescence

Extension of the very short shelf-life of many commercially important plant commodities is highly desirable, and in some cases, critical. Modified atmospheres and removal of ethylene can achieve this effect, as can irradiation. Ripening of bananas is suppressed by irradiation at 0.25–0.35 kGy; the fruit can later be ripened, if necessary, using ethylene. Comparable effects have been observed for mango, papaya, guava, and other tropical and subtropical fruits (IAEA, 1968; Akamine & Moy, 1983; Moy, 1983; Thomas, 1986a). These fruits are susceptible to chilling injury and cannot be held at temperatures below 10–15 °C, so that the availability of an alternative means of extending shelf-life is very attractive.

Various adverse effects may occur in certain fruits exposed to doses exceeding 1 kGy. Detrimental effects on oranges, grapefruit, lemons, limes, bananas, avocados, grapes, olives, figs, cucumbers, summer squash, peppers, artichokes, lettuce, endive, and sweet corn have been reported by a number of investigators (Bramlage & Couey, 1965; Bramlage & Lipton, 1965; Maxie & Abdel-Kader, 1966; Lipton et al., 1967; Maxie et al., 1971; Staden, 1973; Thomas, 1986a,b,c). Sensitivity to chilling injury may also be increased.

Doses exceeding 1 kGy are required for effective suppression of ripening of most temperate zone fruits such as apples, pears, and stone fruits. Such treatment often produces damaging effects, including uneven ripening and softening. The severity of scald on apples may be reduced by doses of 1–2 kGy (Clarke, 1971; Moy, 1983). Chemical scald inhibitors such as diphenylamine and ethoxyquin are effective, but their health effects are currently being reviewed. Irradiation might be a suitable alternative should approval for their use be withdrawn.

Mushrooms have a very short shelf-life. The cap opens, the stem elongates, and the gills darken within 1 day at 10 °C, 2 days at about 4 °C, or 5 days at 0 °C (Thomas, 1988). Staden (1973) reported that treatment with 0.06–1 kGy inhibited cap opening and stalk elongation, and prolonged the shelf-life by up to 1 week. Similar results were reported by Thomas (1988), who found that a dose of about 1 kGy soon after harvest prolonged shelf-life at 10 °C from 1 day to 5–6 days. Most investigators report that sensory quality is unaffected by irradiation. For example, Kovacs & Vas (1974) reported that a panel found no differences in taste in treated mushrooms, either immediately after treatment or after storage.

Avocados are very sensitive to irradiation. Delay of ripening is best accomplished at doses of 0.02–0.1 kGy; higher doses produce skin blemishes and internal discoloration (Thomas, 1986b).

Composition and quality

The calorific value of fresh fruits and vegetables is not reduced by treatment with tolerated doses of ionizing radiation. Insignificant losses of niacin, riboflavin, thiamine, and β-carotene, and somewhat higher losses of vitamin C have been reported (Maxie & Abdel-Kader, 1966). Changes in sugars, fats, proteins, and enzymes are minimal, but changes in pigments can be significant (Romani, 1966; Urbain, 1986).

Doses greater than 0.6 kGy produce solubilization of pectins, cellulose, hemicellulose and starch, resulting in softening of fresh fruits and vegetables. While this is undesirable since it causes difficulties in handling, it can be avoided by processing at low temperature or under an inert atmosphere, or a combination of the two (Maxie & Abdel-Kader, 1966), but the latter reduces the effectiveness with which insects and microorganisms are controlled.

Decay

Post-harvest decay is currently controlled by means of fungicides, reduced-oxygen atmospheres, atmospheres containing some carbon dioxide or carbon monoxide, or treatment with hot water. The minimum dose of ionizing radiation thought to be effective in controlling post-harvest fungi is 1.75 kGy (Sommer & Fortlage, 1966). This is close to the maximum dose of 2.25 kGy that most fresh commodities can tolerate without significant loss of firmness, increased susceptibility to mechanical injury, ripening abnormalities, and altered flavour (Maxie et al., 1971).

Maxie et al. (1971) concluded that strawberries were the only fruit that could be successfully irradiated on a commercial basis in the USA, other fruit being too sensitive to survive the dosage needed for disease control. In South Africa, commercial irradiation of strawberries at a dose of 2 kGy increased shelf-life under refrigeration by about 5 days (Diehl, 1990). A combination of cold storage and a dose of 2.5 kGy has been found to prolong the shelf-life of Dukat strawberries by 9 days (Zegota, 1988). In the USA, strawberries treated using a combination of carbon dioxide and irradiation below 1 kGy have been sold commercially since 1992.

The benefits and limitations of treating fresh fruits and vegetables with ionizing radiation at doses of 2–6 kGy have been summarized by Moy (1983), who concluded that a combination of irradiation and heat treatment was promising, as it took advantage of synergistic effects between the two to achieve pasteurization at lower doses and temperatures.

3.3.2 Nuts and dried fruits and vegetables

The treatment of nuts and dried fruits and vegetables with ionizing radiation is used mainly for purposes of insect disinfestation, but disease-causing microorganisms may also be inactivated and sprouting in nuts inhibited. These commodities may be treated by exposing the finished package to radiation, thus avoiding reinfestation if the package is resistant to insects.

Thomas (1988) reported that exposure of dried fruits to ionizing radiation at doses greater than 4 kGy can reduce toughness, improve rehydration, and shorten cooking time. However, these doses may speed up development of rancidity in tree nuts during storage (Fuller, 1986). The flavour of almonds was unaffected, but pistachios irradiated at 0.6 kGy suffered some flavour effect. Raisins and prunes appear to be unchanged.

3.3.3 Spices

Large numbers of moulds, bacteria, and their heat-resistant spores may be present in natural spices and related materials such as dehydrated vegetable seasonings. Irradiation under good manufacturing conditions can improve the hygienic quality of dehydrated vegetables, spices, herbs, and other dry ingredients (Langerak, 1978; Kiss & Farkas, 1988; Katusin-Razem et al., 1988). These dry products are much less sensitive to ionizing energy than their hydrated counterparts, and losses in quality are not evident even at doses as high as 10 kGy. Soil microorganisms are always present on the growing plant, and increase in number during the drying process. Contaminated seasonings can ultimately lead to spoilage of the foods they are used to flavour. Canned meats may spoil, and severe outbreaks of salmonella poisoning in Canada and Norway were found to have been caused by contaminated pepper (Farkas, 1987). A recent episode of salmonellosis in Sweden was caused by contaminated white pepper (Persson, 1988), while in Germany a ready-to-eat food preparation had to be recalled, at a cost of 30–40 million Marks, because of salmonella contamination of paprika (Anon, 1993).

Ethylene oxide is commonly used to reduce numbers of microorganisms to acceptable levels, but there are concerns regarding the possible mutagenicity and carcinogenicity of its residues, as well as the adverse health effects on the workers. Irradiation is also effective for this purpose and is one of the alternatives to fumigation. For example, irradiation of ground or granulated paprika at 6.5 kGy was more effective than treatment with ethylene oxide over 48 hours in a sterilizing chamber at 25–30 °C (Llorente Franco et al., 1986). Farkas (1983, 1988) and Urbain (1986) reported that doses of 8–20 kGy produced a large reduction in microbiological load. Farkas found no flavour changes in meats prepared using spices treated with a dose of 20 kGy, and no change in the flavour profile of spices dosed at 26 kGy.

In Europe and the United States irradiated spices have been used for some time; the United States permits treatment with doses as high as 30 kGy (FDA regulation, 1992). As a side benefit, any insects that may be present will be destroyed by the high dosages used.

3.3.4 Grains and grain products

The chief problem encountered in grains and grain products is insect infestation. Fumigation with pesticides such as ethylene dibromide, ethylene oxide, methyl bromide, and phosphine is the control method most commonly used. As mentioned earlier, some of these chemicals have been banned in a number of countries. In addition, treatment requires that the grain remain undisturbed for several days and, with certain pesticides, penetration of the commodity may not be uniform, so that some pests may survive and develop resistance. The chemicals are also highly toxic, presenting a hazard to the workers using them. Irradiation is an alternative, and could become the preferred treatment where use of the chemical fumigants is forbidden.

The dosage required for insect control is fairly low, of the order of 1 kGy or less. Commercial irradiation of grain with electron accelerators has been used in the former Soviet Union since 1981 (Diehl, 1990).

Disinfestation is aimed at preventing losses caused by insects in stored grains, pulses, flour, cereals, coffee beans, dried fruits, dried nuts, and other dried food products. Dosages in the range 0.2–0.7 kGy are required, those at the upper end of the range being needed to destroy insects. International activities in the area of insect disinfestation are summarized in the proceedings of a 1983 international conference (Moy, 1985), and by Tilton & Burditt (1983).

Special techniques are needed for grain irradiation, as the commodity is usually stored in sizeable amounts. If electron accelerators are used, the grain must be moved past the accelerator at high speed. X-rays and gamma rays have much greater penetrating power than accelerated electrons, and so thin layers are not needed. Since grains are usually unloaded from ship to dockside through tunnels, all three methods of treatment can be used during the transfer process. Of the three methods, treatment with accelerated electrons is the cheapest for high-volume operations.

3.4 Animal products

3.4.1 Poultry

Poultry is known to be contaminated with many types of bacteria. Removal of the viscera eliminates most of the internal contamination, but the external surfaces and, to a lesser degree, the inner ones may still give relatively high bacterial counts. The shelf-life of refrigerated poultry is in the range 8–17 days, depending on how well sanitary conditions have been maintained during processing.

Both *Salmonella* and *Campylobacter*, which cause human intestinal disease, may exist in the digestive tracts of poultry, livestock, rodents, insects, and wild animals. Of the poultry sold in the United Kingdom, 60–80% may be contaminated with *Salmonella* and up to 100% may contain *Campylobacter* (Roberts, 1990). Subclinical *Salmonella* infection in birds would be extremely difficult to prevent, but most human disease could be avoided by irradiation of finished packages. As with *Salmonella*, the main vehicles for the transmission of *Campylobacter* are poultry and unpasteurized milk (WHO, 1992). Both *Salmonella* and *Campylobacter* are easily destroyed by irradiation, and a number of scientists have recommended it as a way of destroying these and other pathogens in foods of animal origin (Kampelmacher, 1981; Mossel & Stegeman, 1985; WHO, 1987). Other bacteria may also be present in poultry, including *Staphylococcus aureus, Clostridium perfringens, Yersinia enterocolitica*, and *Listeria monocytogenes*.

Prachasitthisakdi et al. (1984) reported that a 4-kGy dose or less was sufficient to inactivate disease-causing organisms in poultry. The FDA recently approved a dose of 3 kGy to control disease-causing organisms in poultry (Food and Drug Administration, 1990). This dosage can also reduce non-spore-forming spoilage bacteria to sufficiently low levels to extend the shelf-life by 1–2 weeks. Nutritional and sensory qualities are not affected by the treatment. Irradiated poultry meat has been sold in a few supermarkets in the USA since September 1993. Ouwerkerk (1981) suggested that salmonellosis in Canada could be addressed effectively by the irradiation of poultry with a dose of 3 kGy. In 1987, a poultry processor in France began commercial irradiation of frozen deboned chicken with an electron accelerator, processing 7000 tonnes per year at a dose of 3 kGy (Wagner & Sillard, 1989).

3.4.2 Meat

Meat such as beef, veal, pork, and lamb is almost always shipped from packing houses to retail stores in bulk form (e.g. sides of beef). The method of preservation used up to that point is refrigeration. The meat is then cut up in the retail store and further preserved by refrigeration (4–5 °C). The shelf-life of the retail product is short (roughly 72 hours), because spoilage is much more rapid in small pieces. Spoilage is caused primarily by microorganisms or chemical processes, the latter essentially by the action of atmospheric oxygen.

Meat is known to be contaminated with various types of pathogens. Most of the spoilage organisms as well as virtually all the pathogenic bacteria may be killed by substerilizing doses of ionizing radiation (analogous to pasteurization), thus extending the shelf-life. Irradiation does not, however, prevent the colour changes or the development of rancidity resulting from oxygen attack, special treatment being needed for this purpose (Urbain, 1973).

Most meat can tolerate higher doses of radiation if precautions are taken. Doses of the order of 25–45 kGy can completely eliminate viable bacteria, yeasts, and moulds (sterilization). Prior to irradiation, autolytic enzymes must be inactivated by heat treatment, and oxygen must be excluded by vacuum packaging in cans or plastic laminates.

Virtually all the work on the sterilization of meat and seafood was carried out by the United States Army between 1953 and 1980 with the aim of making foods available that would remain safe for human consumption in ambient conditions. Among the sterilized products successfully developed were beef, pork, and lamb roasts, beef patties, ham, bacon, pork sausage, cooked salami, chicken, turkey slices, shrimp, and codfish cake.

It is well known in some countries that fresh pork must be cooked thoroughly because it may contain *Trichinella spiralis*. None the less, trichinellosis still occurs, sometimes leading to death. The larvae of the parasite can be rendered noninfective by irradiation with a 0.3-kGy dose. The feasibility of treating pork in this manner to render it "trichinella-safe" has been demonstrated in a programme supported by a trade association and two government agencies in the USA (Brake et al., 1985). Low-dose irradiation could also reduce the risk of cysticercosis, caused by the pork tapeworm (Verster et al., 1977), and toxoplasmosis, caused by *Toxoplasma gondii* (Baldelli et al., 1971; Dubey et al., 1985).

Infections caused by eating undercooked beef containing cysts of the beef tapeworm are seen worldwide, but can be prevented by a 0.4-kGy dose of ionizing energy or by freezing. It also appears that a number of other parasitic protozoa and helminths of great health significance in tropical regions may be killed by low-dose irradiation (1 kGy or less) with no effect on the taste of the food.

3.4.3 Seafood

Seafood has a very limited shelf-life and is particularly difficult to preserve. Many disease-causing organisms have been identified in fish and other seafood. Among those causing problems are *Salmonella, Staphylococcus, Clostridium perfringens*, pathogenic strains of *Escherichia coli* and hepatitis A virus, all of which are found mainly in contaminated inland waters or in improperly handled and stored fish. *Vibrio parahaemolyticus* and *V. vulnificus* are hazards for people who eat raw fish, and *Yersinia enterocolitica* can grow even under refrigeration.

Of great concern is *Clostridium botulinum* type E, the spores of which are more resistant to ionizing radiation than most other spoilage organisms in fish (Eklund, 1982). The recommended dosage for fish suspected of containing this organism is less than 2.2 kGy, a dose which will allow other spoilage organisms to predominate and serve as an indicator of spoilage before type E can develop its toxin. In addition, storage temperatures should be kept below 3.3 °C. *Vibrio cholerae* and *Shigella* may also pose problems in humans and can be controlled by low-dose irradiation.

Disease-causing helminths in shellfish from polluted waters may also give rise to public health problems. In general, low-dose irradiation for seafood consumed raw (such as sashimi) will result in the destruction of parasites, thereby eliminating the major risk associated with the consumption of these foods.

Substerilizing doses of ionizing radiation can substantially prolong the shelf-life of fish and shellfish. Ronsivalli et al. (1969) reported an extension of the shelf-life of cod fillets from 15 days when untreated to 36 days at 0.6 °C by exposure to 1.5 kGy. Ampola & Ronsivalli (1969) reported that the shelf-life of eviscerated haddock decreased with increasing time on the ship before processing with ionizing radiation. This suggests that fish should be treated as soon as possible after being caught.

Treatment of codfish, clams, haddock, and herring with shipboard ionizing radiation doubled or tripled their shelf-lives (Carver et al., 1969). The shelf-life of eviscerated haddock was also extended by shipboard irradiation, but this was not true for redfish (Ehlermann & Reinacher, 1978).

Vibrio parahaemolyticus, V. vulnificus and hepatitis A virus are common pathogenic contaminants of fish and shellfish. Recent reports indicate that consumption of raw or improperly cooked contaminated molluscs and crustaceans has led to sickness and high fatality rates. In 1983, *Shigella* was implicated in the deaths of 14 people in the Netherlands (Farkas, 1987). Frozen shrimps are now commercially irradiated in Belgium, France and the Netherlands.

A great deal of interest has been shown in northern Europe in extending the shelf-life and reducing the hygienic risks of European brown shrimps, which are small, and have defied successful use of peeling machines. Peeling is therefore carried out mainly in private houses and, because of the time taken to transport them to the houses, the useful shelf-life is reduced. Contamination of the shrimps with pathogenic organisms is unavoidable and chemical preservatives are generally used to avoid problems. Research in several European countries has shown that irradiation of the peeled shrimps with a 1.3-kGy dose gave far better results than chemical preservation in terms of reducing microorganism counts and maintaining low counts for longer periods. In addition, no pathogenic staphylococci were found in the irradiated samples, compared with high counts in the untreated and chemically preserved samples (Ehlermann & Münzner, 1976).

3.4.4 Eggs

Poultry infected with *Salmonella* may lay contaminated eggs. Cases of salmonellosis in the United States have been identified as having been caused by the consumption of infected eggs (St Louis et al., 1988), and similar cases have been reported from many other countries.

Morgan & Siu (1957) reported that 3–6-kGy doses could kill salmonellae in whole eggs and egg magma, and in the 1960s, the United States Army reported that 5-kGy doses could destroy salmonellae in frozen shelled eggs and powdered eggs. In a recent review, Farkas (1987) reported that a 2-kGy dose in air would reduce salmonella counts in egg powder or egg yolk solids by up to 1000-fold with no loss of sensory qualities or nutritional content. Powdered eggs are currently being treated with ionizing radiation in the Netherlands to control salmonella (Diehl, 1990).

Irradiation of shell eggs to control *Salmonella* may not be technically feasible as the dose required (2–4 kGy) may adversely affect a number of characteristics of the eggs, e.g. thinning the egg white or weakening the yolk membrane (Urbain, 1986). Harewood (1992), on the other hand, reported that there was no significant difference in the sensory characteristics of soft-boiled eggs between control eggs and those irradiated with either 1.5 or 3.0 kGy and stored at 4 °C for 25 days. A significant difference was found, however, in the sensory characteristics of eggs irradiated with 3.0 kGy and control eggs when fried or scrambled.

3.4.5 Dairy products

Many dairy products may develop objectionable changes in flavour, odour, and colour when irradiated, even at doses as low as 0.5 kGy (Urbain, 1986). Camembert cheese made from raw milk, however, can be successfully irradiated with a dose of up to 2.5 kGy to control *Listeria monocytogenes* (Bougle & Stahl, 1993). In France, irradiation of Camembert cheese has been approved and a commercial irradiator has been designed specifically for this purpose.

3.5 Combination processes

Ionizing radiation alone may not always be sufficient to achieve the intended effect; the dose required may produce undesirable results, or the cost may be too great. The desired result may, however, be achieved with a combination of irradiation and some other treatment.

Obvious examples are irradiation in combination with refrigeration or heating, both of which reduce the dose of ionizing radiation required, thereby reducing the cost and preserving the quality of the product. Vacuum packaging and irradiation are another effective combination useful for prolonging shelf-life. Reducing the water content of a food, which has a preservative effect, will also render treatment with ionizing radiation more effective.

Effective combinations of chemical treatment and irradiation are available, such as the use of salt, which reduces water activity, and of nitrite, which can prevent the production of botulinus toxin. Carbon dioxide can both increase the acidity of foods and prevent *Clostridium botulinum* from producing toxin.

3.6 Summary and conclusions

In conventional food processing, a number of physical and chemical techniques are used to preserve foods, temperature regulation also playing an important role. Food irradiation should be viewed as another tool available to supplement the more traditional means of food preservation. Insects, parasites and most disease-causing microorganisms in foods may be effectively deactivated by exposure to relatively low doses of ionizing radiation. The shelf-life of many foods may be increased, often sufficiently to make products acceptable to humans that would otherwise have to be diverted for use as animal feed or destroyed. Sterilization techniques are sometimes available, allowing food to be stored indefinitely at ambient temperatures.

Most low-dosage radiation of fresh fruits and vegetables produces an extended shelf-life without materially affecting quality and sensory attributes. Control of microbial populations often requires higher doses, leading to adverse effects such as mushiness and discoloration. In such cases, however, combination treatments may well produce the desired effects.

The shelf-life of animal products may be increased by treatment with low-dose ionizing radiation in conjunction with refrigeration. Sterilizing doses must generally be applied in the absence of oxygen and when meat is frozen to avoid unpleasant tastes and odours. A preliminary blanching is also needed to inactivate enzymes that would cause undesirable effects.

Other applications include: the inhibition of sprouting; increasing the hydration rate of dehydrated vegetables; increasing the drying rate of fruits; reducing the cooking time of some vegetables; reducing the level of sodium nitrite needed to cure meat; and tenderizing beef. Sterilization of certain foods has led to a number of benefits in terms of long-term product storage.

Many foods treated with ionizing radiation have not encountered acceptability problems, but others have exhibited highly undesirable side-effects. It should be noted, however, that heat-treatment of food often produces more serious deficiencies. Most end-products of irradiation fall somewhere between these two extremes; practicality and economics will dictate whether useful, everyday applications will ultimately emerge worldwide.

References

Adesuyi SA, Mackenzie JA (1973) The inhibition of sprouting in stored yams, *Dioscorea rotunda* poir, by gamma radiation and chemicals. In: *Radiation preservation of food. Proceedings of a symposium held in Bombay, November 1972*, Vienna, International Atomic Energy Agency, pp. 127–136.

Akamine EK, Moy JH (1983) Delay in postharvest ripening and senescence of fruits. In: Josephson ES, Peterson MS, eds. *Preservation of food by ionizing radiation*, Vol. 3. Boca Raton, FL, CRC Press, pp. 129–158.

Ampola VG, Ronsivalli LJ (1969) Effect of pre-irradiation quality of eviscerated haddock on postirradiation shelf-life of fillets. *Journal of food science*, **34**: 27–30.

Anon (1993) Paprika recall. *International food safety news*, **2**: 99.

Baldelli B et al. (1971) [Effects of gamma radiation on a strain of *Toxoplasma* isolated from dog.] *Parasitologia*, **13**:105 (in Italian).

Bougle D, Stahl V (1993) Éradication de bactéries pathogènes (*Listeria monocytogenes* et *Salmonella*) de Camembert au lait cru par rayonnements ionisants. In: *Cost-benefit aspects of food irradiation*. Vienna, International Atomic Energy Agency.

Brake RJ et al. (1985) Destruction of *Trichinella spiralis* by low-dose irradiation of infected pork. *Journal of food safety*, **7**:127–143.

Bramlage WJ, Couey HM (1965) *Gamma radiation of fruits to extend market life*. Washington, DC, US Department of Agriculture (Marketing Research Report 717).

Bramlage WJ, Lipton WJ (1965) *Gamma radiation of vegetables to extend market life*. Washington, DC, US Department of Agriculture (Marketing Research Report 703).

Burditt AK Jr (1982) Food irradiation as a quarantine treatment of fruits. *Food technology*, **36**:51–54, 58–60, 62.

Carver JH et al. (1969) Irradiation of fish at sea. In: Kreuzer R, ed. *Freezing and irradiation of fish*. London, Fishing News (Books).

CAST (1989) *Ionizing energy in food processing and pest control. II. Applications*. Ames, IA, Council for Agricultural Science and Technology (Report No. 1159).

Clarke ID (1971) Effects of radiation treatments. In: Hulme AC, ed. *The biochemistry of fruits and their products*, Vol. 2. New York, Academic Press.

Couey HM (1983) Development of quarantine systems for host fruits of the medfly. *Horticultural science*, **18**:45–47.

Curzio OA, Croci CA (1983) Extending onion storage life by gamma-irradiation. *Journal of food processing and preservation*, **7**:19–23.

Diehl JF (1990) *Safety of irradiated food*. New York, Marcel Dekker.

Dubey JP et al. (1985) Effect of irradiation on the viability of *Toxoplasma gondii* cysts in tissues of mice and pigs. *Journal of the American Veterinary Medical Association*, **187**:304.

Ehlermann D, Münzner R (1976) [Radiation preservation of North Sea shrimps.] *Archiv für Lebensmittelhygiene*, **27**:50–55 (in German).

Ehlermann D, Reinacher E (1978) Some conclusions from shipboard experiments on the radurization of whole fish in the Federal Republic of Germany. In: *Food preservation by irradiation*, Vol. I. Vienna, International Atomic Energy Agency, pp. 321–331 (IAEA-SM-221/18).

Eklund MW (1982) Significance of *Clostridium botulinum* in fishery products preserved short of sterilization. *Food technology*, **36**:107–112.

Farkas J (1983) Radurization and radicidation: spices. In: Josephson ES, Peterson MS, eds. *Preservation of food by ionizing radiation*, Vol. 3. Boca Raton, FL, CRC Press, pp. 109–128.

Farkas J (1987) Decontamination, including parasite control, of dried, chilled, and frozen foods by irradiation. *Acta alimentaria*, **16**:351–384.

Farkas J (1988) *Irradiation of dry food ingredients*. Boca Raton, FL, CRC Press.

FDA regulation (1992) 21 Code of Federal Regulation 179, 26.

Food and Drug Administration (1990) Irradiation of poultry. *Federal register*, **55**:18538.

Fuller G (1986) *Quality evaluation of irradiated dried fruits and tree nuts*. Washington, DC, US Department of Energy, Energy Technology Division (Interagency Agreement No. DE-A104-83AL24327).

Goresline HE et al. (1964) Tentative classification of food irradiation processes with microbiological objectives. *Nature*, **204**:237–238.

Grünewald T (1978) Studies on sprout inhibition of onions by irradiation in the Federal Republic of Germany. In: *Food preservation by irradiation. Proceedings of a Symposium held in Wageningen, November 1977*. Vienna, International Atomic Energy Agency, p. 123–131.

Harewood PM (1992) *Technological assessment of irradiated eggs*. West Kingston, University of Rhode Island (Ph.D. dissertation)

IAEA (1968) *Preservation of fruits and vegetables by radiation. Proceedings of the Joint FAO/IAEA Panel, Vienna, 1–5 August 1966*. Vienna, International Atomic Energy Agency (Publication No. STI/PUB/149).

IAEA (1973) *Radiation preservation of food. Proceedings of a symposium, Bombay, India, 1972*. Vienna, International Atomic Energy Agency (Publication No. STI/PUB/470).

Kader AA (1986) Potential applications of ionizing radiation in postharvest handling of fresh fruits and vegetables. *Food technology* **40**:117–121.

Kampelmacher EH (1981) Prospects of eliminating pathogens by the process of food irradiation. In: *Combination processes in food irradiation. Proceedings of a symposium held in Colombo, November 1980*. Vienna, International Atomic Energy Agency, pp. 265–289.

Katusin-Razem B et al. (1988) Radiation decontamination of tea herbs. *Journal of food science*, **53**:1120–1126.

Kiss I, Farkas J (1988) Irradiation as a method for decontamination of spices. *Food reviews international*, **4**:77–92.

Kovacs E, Vas K (1974) Effects of ionizing radiations on some organoleptic characteristics of edible mushrooms. *Acta alimentaria*, **3**:11–17.

Kwon JH et al. (1985) Effects of gamma irradiation dose and timing of treatment after harvest on the storability of garlic bulbs. *Journal of food science*, **50**:379–381.

Langerak DI (1978) The influence of irradiation and packaging on the quality of prepacked vegetables. *Annales de la nutrition et de l'alimentation*, **32**:569–586.

Lipton WJ et al. (1967) Conclusions about radiation. In: *United fresh fruit and vegetable yearbook*. Washington, DC, United Fresh Fruit and Vegetable Association, pp. 173–174, 176, 178, 181.

Llorente Franco S et al. (1986) Effectiveness of ethylene oxide and gamma irradiation on the microbiological population of three types of paprika. *Journal of food science*, **51**:1571–1572.

Lu JY et al. (1986) Effects of gamma radiation on nutritive and sensory qualities of sweet potato storage roots. *Journal of food quality*, **9**:425–435.

Matsuyama A, Umeda K (1983) Sprout inhibition in tubers and bulbs. In: Josephson ES, Peterson MS, eds. *Preservation of food by ionizing radiation*, Vol. 3. Boca Raton, FL, CRC Press, pp. 159–213.

Maxie EC, Abdel-Kader AS (1966) Food irradiation — physiology of fruits as related to feasibility of the technology. *Advances in food research*, **15**:105–145.

Maxie EC et al. (1971) Infeasibility of irradiating fresh fruits and vegetables. *Horticultural science*, **6**:202–204.

Morgan BH, Siu RGH (1957) Action of ionizing radiation in individual foods. In: Bailey SD et al., eds. *Radiation preservation of food*. Washington, DC, US Government Printing Office, pp. 268–294.

Mossel DAA, Stegeman H (1985) Irradiation: an effective mode of processing food for safety. In: *Food irradiation processing. Proceedings of a symposium held in Washington, DC, 1985*. Vienna, International Atomic Energy Agency, p. 251.

Moy JH (1983) Radurization and radicidation: fruits and vegetables. In: Josephson ES, Peterson MS, eds. *Preservation of food by ionizing radiation*, Vol. 3. Boca Raton, FL, CRC Press, pp. 83–108.

Moy JH, ed. (1985) *Radiation disinfestation of food and agricultural products. Proceedings of an International Conference held in Honolulu, Hawaii, November 1983*. Honolulu, Hawaii Institute of Tropical Agriculture and Human Resources, University of Hawaii at Manoa.

Ouwerkerk T (1981) Salmonella control in poultry through the use of gamma irradiation. In: *Combination processes in food irradiation. Proceedings of a symposium held in Colombo, November 1980*. Vienna, International Atomic Energy Agency, p. 335–345.

Persson L (1988) [Warning against unirradiated spices!] *Läkartidningen*, **85**:2641 (in Swedish).

Prachasitthisakdi Y et al. (1984) Lethality and flora shift of the psychrotropic and mesophilic bacterial association of frozen shrimps and chicken after radicidation. In: Kiss I, Deak T, Incze K, eds. *Microbial associations and interactions in food*. Budapest, Publishing House of the Hungarian Academy of Sciences, pp. 417–428.

Roberts D (1990) Sources of infection: food. *Lancet*, **336**:859–861.

Romani RJ (1966) Radiobiological parameters in the irradiation of fruits and vegetables. *Advances in food research*, **15**:57–103.

Ronsivalli LJ et al. (1969) Studies in petition-oriented aspects of radiation pasteurization of fishery products. In: *Preservation of fish by irradiation*. Vienna, International Atomic Energy Agency, pp. 1–11 (Publication No. STI/PUB/196).

Sommer NF, Fortlage RJ (1966) Ionizing radiation for control of postharvest diseases of fruits and vegetables. *Advances in food research*, **15**:147–193.

St Louis ME et al. (1988) The emergence of grade A eggs as a major source of *Salmonella enteritidis* infections. *Journal of the American Medical Association*, **259**:2103–2107.

Staden OL (1973) A review of the potential of fruit and vegetable irradiation. *Scientia horticulturae*, **1**:291–308.

Thomas P (1984a) Radiation preservation of foods of plant origin. Part I. Potatoes and other tuber crops. *CRC critical reviews in food science and nutrition*, **19**:327–370.

Thomas P (1984b) Radiation preservation of foods of plant origin. Part II. Onions and other bulb crops. *CRC critical reviews in food science and nutrition*, **21**:95–136.

Thomas P (1986a) Radiation preservation of foods of plant origin. Part III. Bananas, mangoes, and papayas. *CRC critical reviews in food science and nutrition*, **23**:147–205.

Thomas P (1986b) Radiation preservation of foods of plant origin. Part IV. Subtropical fruits: citrus, grapes, and avocados. *CRC critical reviews in food science and nutrition*, **24**:53–89.

Thomas P (1986c) Radiation preservation of foods of plant origin. Part V. Temperate fruits: pome fruits, stone fruits, and berries. *CRC critical reviews in food science and nutrition*, **24**:357–400.

Thomas P (1988) Radiation preservation of foods of plant origin. Part VI. Mushrooms, tomatoes, minor fruits and vegetables, dried fruits, and nuts. *CRC critical reviews in food science and nutrition*, **26**:313–358.

Tilton EW, Burditt AK Jr (1983) Insect disinfestation of grain and fruit. In: Josephson ES, Peterson MS, eds. *Preservation of food by ionizing radiation,* Vol. 3. Boca Raton, FL, CRC Press, pp. 215–229.

Urbain WM (1973) The low-dose radiation preservation of retail cuts of meat. In: *Radiation preservation of food*. Vienna, International Atomic Energy Agency, pp. 505–521 (Publication No. STI/PUB/317).

Urbain WM (1978) Food irradiation. *Advances in food research*, **24**:155–227.

Urbain WM (1986) *Food irradiation*. New York, Academic Press.

Verster A et al. (1977) The eradication of tapeworms in pork and beef carcasses by irradiation. *Radiation physics and chemistry*, **9**:769–773.

Wagner J, Sillard M (1989) Pasteurizing with electrons. *Food engineering international*, **14**(2):38–41.

WHO (1987) *Task Force Meeting on the use of irradiation to ensure hygienic quality of food, Vienna, Austria, 1986*. Geneva, World Health Organization (unpublished document WHO/EHE/FOS/87.2; available on request from Food Safety, World Health Organization, 1211 Geneva 27, Switzerland).

WHO (1988) *Food irradiation. A technique for preserving and improving the safety of food*. Geneva, World Health Organization.

WHO (1992) *WHO Commission on Health and Environment: report of the Panel on Food and Agriculture*. Geneva, World Health Organization (unpublished document, WHO/EHE/92.2).

Zegota H (1988) Suitability of Dukat strawberries for studying effects on shelf life of irradiation combined with cold storage. *Zeitschrift für Lebensmittel-Untersuchung und -Forschung*, **187**:111–114.

4.
Chemistry of food irradiation

4.1 Introduction

In this chapter, the key features of the chemistry of food irradiation are reviewed; for further information, see Diehl (1990) and Food and Drug Administration (1980). The latter, though less recent, contains a good summary of the critical chemical factors that should be considered in assessing the safety of irradiated foods.

4.2 Background radiation and induced radioactivity

All foods are radioactive to some extent, albeit at very low levels. People are also exposed to background radiation from outer space and from naturally occurring radioactive elements in soil, rocks, and the atmosphere. The health effects of background radiation can be estimated by extrapolation from those of known exposures to high doses. On this basis, background radiation is estimated to cause 0.3–1% of all cancers in humans (CAST, 1986), but this is believed to be an overestimate of the true effect.

Short-lived radioactivity can be induced in some foods if the energy level of the radiation is sufficiently high (greater than 14 MeV with electron beams). Consequently, the Joint FAO/IAEA/WHO Expert Committee on the Wholesomeness of Irradiated Foods conservatively recommended 10 MeV as the maximum permissible energy for electron generators, and 5 MeV for X-rays (WHO, 1965, 1981). (The figure for X-rays was set at a lower level because they are more efficient in inducing radioactivity than electrons of the same energy). Below these maxima, induced radioactivity has never been observed in foods treated with doses up to 50 kGy (Diehl, 1990). The energy level produced by cobalt-60 and caesium-137 is not high enough to cause radioactivity.

The Codex Alimentarius Commission (FAO, 1984), the Advisory Committee on Irradiated and Novel Foods (1986), and the Food and Drug Administration (1986) have all adopted 10 MeV as the maximum for electron beams and 5 MeV for X-rays, as have the governments of most countries that permit food irradiation. In its final rule of 18 April 1986, the FDA stated that no evidence had been submitted to contradict its finding that irradiation of food does not cause it to become radioactive (Food and Drug Administration, 1986).

It has been estimated on theoretical grounds that the maximum level set by the Joint Committee would result in an induced radioactivity so low that human cancers would be increased by only $0.3–1 \times 10^{-8}\%$, which may be compared with the estimate of 0.3–1% from natural background radiation previously mentioned (CAST, 1986). Terry & McColl (1992) calculated theoretical levels of induced radioactivity using semi-empirical formulae, and concluded that the induced activities in a wide range of foods less than 24 hours after irradiation were well below the level judged to be worthy of concern. Irradiation in the commercially useful range will therefore not generate measurable radioactivity in foods.

4.3 Types of radiation and their effects

The electromagnetic spectrum encompasses the very short-wavelength cosmic rays, gamma rays, X-rays, the ultraviolet, visible and infrared regions, microwaves, radar, and finally, the very low-energy, long wavelengths associated with the communication bands. Visible light can break only the weakest intramolecular bonds, ultraviolet light somewhat stronger bonds, while X-rays and gamma rays are sufficiently powerful to expel orbiting electrons from atoms to produce free radicals. This comparatively high-energy form of radiation is called ionizing radiation, and is produced by X-ray generators, electron accelerators, and decaying radionuclides. Gamma rays from cobalt-60 have been most widely used in the past. Electron accelerators and X-ray converters may, however, play a much more important role in the future. Gamma rays penetrate foodstuffs deeply because of their relatively short wavelengths.

The total amount of ionizing radiation absorbed by a food represents the radiation dose. In food irradiation, even the largest doses result in a very low level of absorbed energy. For example, if all the energy absorbed by a food given a 10-kGy dose were converted into heat energy, the temperature of the food would rise by only $2.4°C$ (assuming that the food has the heat capacity of water).

As previously mentioned, the concentration of radiolytic products generated usually increases linearly with the radiation dose. The radiolytic products formed are essentially the same whether the food is exposed to large or small amounts of radiation. Dose-rate effects, as opposed to those related to dose, are seldom important in food-irradiation processes.

As the amount of energy absorbed from the radiation increases, the first effect will be the formation of excited molecules. These may then undergo de-excitation (a reversal of the process) or receive additional energy, which leads to dissociation or ionization. Chemical bonds are broken and either neutral or electrically charged free radicals are produced; these are almost always unstable, extremely reactive chemical entities. Secondary effects involving such highly reactive free radicals may include reactions leading to recombination, dimerization, disproportionation, and electron capture. As a result, a very complicated mixture of stable end-products is possible. While the primary effects are generally nonspecific, secondary effects depend to a large extent on the particular chemical structures involved and on the nature and concentration of other compounds.

Free radicals may thus be formed either directly by reaction with high-energy electrons, or indirectly by interaction with hydroxyl radicals (·OH), hydrogen atoms (·H) or low-energy solvated electrons. The last three species are produced by the radiolysis of water and are the primary initiating agents responsible for the formation of most of the resulting radiolysis products. Thus, the percentage of water in a given food and the degree of hydration of various food molecules have a profound effect on the magnitude and nature of the radiolysis products formed.

The vast majority of free radicals are extremely short-lived, reacting almost instantaneously to form stable chemical entities. However, in foods that are deep-frozen or exist as dry solids, diffusion is limited, and it is then not uncommon for free radicals to persist for a long time. For example, free radicals trapped in bones or seafood shells may persist for months or even years.

4.4 Water

With few exceptions, water is a major component of foods, the water content ranging from about 90% in vegetables, 80% in fruits and 60% in meat, to 40% in bread. Even so-called dry foods, such as wheat flour and dried vegetables, contain considerable amounts of water. The effects of irradiation on water are thus obviously extremely important. Water forms a number of radiolytic products, including hydroxyl radicals (·OH), hydrated electrons ($e^-_{H_2O}$ or e^-_{aq}), hydrogen atoms (·H), hydrogen molecules (H_2), hydrogen peroxide (H_2O_2), and hydrated protons (H_3O^+), each of which may react with food components.

The only stable end-products of water radiolysis are hydrogen and hydrogen peroxide, which are largely lost prior to consumption. Thus, even where radiation doses are high, the final concentrations of these two products are very low. Hydrogen peroxide is an oxidizing agent, but is of much less importance than the highly reactive short-lived radical and hydrated electron intermediates. The hydroxyl radical is a powerful oxidizing agent, while the hydrated electron is a strong reducing agent. Hydrogen atoms are slightly weaker reducing agents. As a result, both oxidation and reduction reactions take place when foods containing water are irradiated.

In dilute aqueous solutions, both direct and indirect effects may occur, the latter involving the very reactive species formed by the radiolysis of water; they therefore overshadow the direct effects under such conditions. It follows that the destruction suffered by substances in aqueous solution as a result of irradiation is much greater than that of dry materials, where direct effects predominate.

4.5 Dilution

The degradation of solutes depends markedly on the number of reactive radicals present. The more dilute the solution, the greater the chances that solute molecules will find reactive radicals with which to interact. The increasing sensitivity of the solute to radiation with increasing dilution is known as the *dilution effect*. The destruction of a solute can therefore be reduced by irradiating at higher concentrations, as demonstrated in the deactivation of horseradish peroxidases (Delincée & Radola, 1974). Destruction can also be reduced by irradiating the solute of interest in the presence of other solutes which compete for the free radical intermediates of the solvent (Proctor et al., 1952).

4.6 Multicomponent systems

Many investigators have predicted that irradiation will cause major destruction of a large number of important food components. These predictions are based primarily on experiments carried out on pure solutions of individual food components. Foods are multicomponent mixtures, however, and the destruction by irradiation is therefore distributed among most of the components, generally resulting in minimal damage to any one component. Irradiation experiments carried out on foods themselves have shown that the damage is small when the dose is in the acceptable range (Diehl, 1990).

4.7 Oxygen

In equilibrium with air, water contains small amounts of dissolved oxygen, a substance which plays a major role in radiation-mediated reactions. Oxygen can be reduced by hydrogen atoms to the hydroperoxy radical ($\cdot HO_2$), a mild oxidizing agent, which is in equilibrium with the superoxide radical ($\cdot O_2^-$); the latter can also be produced by the reaction of solvated electrons with oxygen. Both the superoxide and hydroperoxy radicals can produce hydrogen peroxide. Reactions such as these consume oxygen, so that an anaerobic matrix may be produced by electron irradiation at high dose rates. However, gamma sources deliver a much lower dose rate, giving oxygen the time to diffuse back into the system. As a result, anaerobic conditions are not usually encountered in gamma irradiation unless the food is irradiated under an inert gas or in a vacuum.

4.8 pH

Many equilibrium reactions are pH-dependent. The nature of the radiolytic products formed may therefore be influenced by the acidity or alkalinity of the reaction medium.

4.9 Temperature

Temperature may have profound effects on the radiolytic products formed. In frozen foods, for example, the reactive intermediates produced from water are trapped and cannot readily react with each other or with the substrate. When the food is warmed, the intermediates characteristically react with each other and not with the substrate so that, when the food again reaches ambient temperature, the damage to the substrate is much less than would have occurred if the food had been irradiated at that temperature to begin with. The irradiation of deep-frozen meat, for example, produces much smaller effects on taste than that of meat at ambient temperatures.

4.10 Radiolytic products

The intensive investigations of the chemistry of food irradiation have to a large extent focused on the nature of the radiolytic products generated. Foods are extremely complex mixtures of chemicals, usually containing hundreds of thousands of different compounds in a wide range of concentrations. Consequently, the complete chemical characterization of any food, whether irradiated or not, is virtually impossible. Thus, while the information contained in the scientific literature is insufficient to enable all the reaction products present in an irradiated food to be completely identified and quantified, it does nevertheless indicate the nature of the radiation chemistry likely to occur in foods.

4.11 Effects on major food constituents

The three major food constituents are carbohydrates, lipids, and proteins, each of which will be considered in turn. Radiation effects have been found in all of them but, even at doses as high as 50 kGy, are so small that it took many years of research to develop analytical methods capable of detecting and characterizing them.

4.11.1 Carbohydrates

In aqueous systems, carbohydrates react primarily with hydroxyl radicals to form ketones, aldehydes, or acids as end-products; deoxygenation may also occur. Glucose alone has been found to generate at least 34 radiolytic products (von Sonntag, 1980). In the presence of oxygen, the yield of deoxy products is decreased, but those of sugar acids and keto sugars are increased. Acid formation leads to significant reduction in pH.

Irradiated starch degrades to dextrins, maltose, and glucose, leading to a decrease in the viscosity of polysaccharides in solution. Advantage has been taken of this in the development of detection methods for irradiated foods (see Chapter 5). Irradiation of maize starch in an aqueous system produces a number of sugars, aldehydes, ketones, alcohols, acids, and peroxides (Dauphin & Saint-Lèbe, 1977). Generally speaking, the amount of water present markedly influences the nature and yield of the products formed. Carbohydrates present as food components are much less prone to degradation than when irradiated in their pure form.

4.11.2 Proteins

Proteins consist of chains of amino acids connected by peptide linkages. An appreciation of the major effects of irradiation on proteins therefore requires an understanding of the reactions undergone by amino acids following irradiation in the presence of water, including the abstraction of hydrogen atoms, reductive deamination, disproportionation, decarboxylation, and reactions between the intermediates formed with the highly reactive products of water radiolysis. The presence of oxygen does not materially change the nature of the radiolytic products formed, although yields are affected.

Proteins may contain about 20 amino acids so that, in combination with the various reactive species produced by the radiolysis of water, a large number of different end-products are possible. In an actual food matrix, the amino acids contained in proteins are less accessible and therefore less susceptible to attack. In addition, radicals formed by the irradiation process are comparatively immobile and are thus much more prone to recombination, as opposed to reaction with other components of the food matrix.

Degradation of proteins to smaller polypeptides can occur as a result of the splitting of carbon–nitrogen bonds and disulfide bridges. Conversely, globular proteins irradiated in solution may undergo aggregation reactions, producing higher relative molecular mass proteins and thus solutions of higher viscosity. Aggregation reactions may also take place when meat is irradiated (Radola, 1974; Uzunov et al., 1972).

Enzymes present in foods are quite stable on irradiation. As a result, irradiation-sterilized food, even if it does not spoil microbiologically, will spoil enzymatically. Thus, foods intended for long-term storage must also be heat-treated to prevent enzymatic spoilage.

There is some evidence to show that radiation damage to the amino acids in proteins is quite limited, little change in amino acid composition generally being observed at doses below 50 kGy. The amino acid composition of codfish, for example, is largely unaffected by radiation (Underdal et al., 1973).

More detailed accounts of some of the effects of irradiation on proteins and amino acids may be found in Diehl et al. (1979), Liebster & Kopoldova (1964), Delincée & Radola (1975), Urbain (1977), Delincée (1983), Simic (1983), and Taub (1983).

4.11.3 Lipids

Since triglycerides comprise the bulk of the lipid portion of foods (generally about 90% or higher), only triglyceride chemistry will be described here.

In contrast to the radiation chemistry of carbohydrates and proteins, where water plays a major role, that of fat is essentially nonaqueous in character since triglycerides are virtually insoluble in water.

The direct effect of radiation on lipids is the production of cation radicals and molecules in the excited state. The main initial reaction of cation radicals is deprotonation, followed by dimerization or disproportionation. Attachment of electrons also occurs, followed by dissociation and decarbonylation or dimerization.

Excited triglycerides can also undergo a wide variety of reactions. A large number of reaction products can therefore be formed, including fatty acids, propanediol and propenediol esters, aldehydes, ketones, diglycerides, di-esters, alkanes and alkenes, methyl esters, hydrocarbons, and shorter-chain triglycerides; for further information, see Delincée (1983).

Vegetable oils have been studied extensively by Nawar and co-workers (Kavalam & Nawar, 1969). Many volatile radiolytic products, including hydrocarbons, aldehydes, and methyl and ethyl esters, have been identified. Other reports (Nawar, 1977, 1983, 1986) describe numerous studies carried out on other lipids. Merritt and co-workers (Merritt & Taub, 1983; Vajdi & Merritt, 1985) have also carried out detailed studies.

All the studies referred to above were carried out under anaerobic conditions. It is believed that irradiation in the presence of oxygen will lead to more rapid auto-oxidation, but this effect has not been extensively studied.

There is little evidence so far to suggest that aromatic or heterocyclic rings are formed, or that existing aromatic rings undergo condensation. Obviously, the formation of either aromatic or heterocyclic ring compounds would be a cause for concern, since some of them would probably be potentially carcinogenic. This is in marked contrast with the ring compounds known to be formed via the cooking process, such as benzo[a]pyrene, a known carcinogen and typical of the polynuclear aromatic hydrocarbons produced by cooking, and the imidazo quinolines, typical of the heterocyclic ring compounds also produced.

In meats, oxidative changes in lipids appear to be small. It is believed that proteins, or protein–carbohydrate interaction products, have an antioxidant effect which increases with radiation dose. These components may therefore serve to mitigate oxidative changes in lipids; there is also some evidence that irradiated meats possess increased oxidative stability (Green & Watts, 1966; Diehl, 1982).

4.11.4 Vitamins

Studies of the effects of irradiation on vitamins have led to differing conclusions depending on whether pure solutions or actual food matrices were investigated. Losses in pure solution are usually far greater. Thus aqueous solutions of vitamin B_1 showed a 50% loss at a dose of 0.5 kGy but, at the same dose, dried whole egg lost less than 5% (Diehl, 1975). Again, this difference may be attributed to the protective action of other food components. In some products, measurements of vitamin content immediately after irradiation may seriously underestimate losses, as degradation may well continue in storage, especially when oxygen is not excluded, as with vitamin E in rolled oats (Diehl, 1979). Irradiation may perhaps also lead to increased vitamin loss during cooking. Losses such as these, however, can be greatly reduced if the food is treated under anaerobic conditions.

Losses of vitamins are not necessarily increased by irradiation and cooking; the effect will vary greatly from vitamin to vitamin and possibly from food to food. In cod, nicotinic acid and riboflavin were little affected, while thiamine losses were over 50% (Kennedy & Ley, 1971). In some cases, the combination of irradiation and cooking may reduce losses, since cooking times for certain foods may be considerably shorter after irradiation; for example, red gram retained more riboflavin, nicotinic acid, and thiamine after irradiation at 10 kGy followed by cooking (Sreenivasan, 1974).

A combination of low temperature and anaerobic conditions is apparently capable of protecting thiamine and vitamin E, which may otherwise suffer great losses during irradiation (Diehl, 1979). The process developed by the United States Army Natick Laboratories for the radiation sterilization of meat at $-30\,°C$ in the absence of oxygen resulted in reduced losses of thiamine in pork as compared with heat-sterilized meat (Thomas et al., 1981).

Ascorbic acid (vitamin C) has been widely studied in a variety of foods (Proctor & O'Meara, 1951; Jensen, 1960; Galetto et al., 1979; Romani et al., 1963; Nagay & Moy, 1985; Moshonas & Shaw, 1984; Beyers & Thomas, 1979; Thomas et al., 1971; Zegota, 1988; Wills, 1965). At practical dose levels for irradiation of fruit and vegetables (1 kGy or less), little vitamin C is lost. The effect of radiation on vitamins is discussed in more detail in Chapter 8.

4.11.5 Conclusions

Carbohydrates, proteins and fats in food matrices are affected only to a small extent by irradiation. Some vitamins, however, are prone to degradation depending on the food type and the conditions of irradiation and storage. To put this in perspective, each food must be considered in terms of its dietary importance. For example, extensive vitamin loss in spices would be of no concern, as they make up a very small part of the total diet. Conversely, meats make up a large part of the diet for many people, and significant losses of vitamins from meat could not easily be tolerated.

4.12 Total yield of radiolytic products

The total yield of radiolytic products is related mainly to the magnitude of the absorbed radiation dose, but certain other factors may affect both the yield and the type of product formed. As mentioned earlier, these include food temperature, viscosity, composition, and environment. These can usually be controlled so as to avoid the formation of less desirable end-products.

Investigations at the Natick laboratory have shown that the radiolytic products formed from beef, chicken, and pork lipid fractions are essentially the same (Food and Drug Administration, 1980). The proportion of fat in the irradiated meat was the determining factor in the amount of radiolytic products formed. Cross-over reaction products were present only in small amounts because reactions between the lipid-derived and protein-derived free radicals can take place only at the interfaces between the tissue phases in meat. This compartmentalization of food components limits the variety of reaction products likely to be produced in foods. As a consequence, irradiated foods of similar composition will probably contain similar reaction products, and such foods may thus be evaluated generically.

The FDA has estimated that, at a radiation dose of 1 kGy, the yield of all reaction products (assuming an average relative molecular mass of 300) will be 30 mg/kg (Food and Drug Administration, 1980). For higher dose levels, as stated above, the yield would be expected to increase linearly.

4.13 Unique radiolytic products

Many of the reaction products referred to in the previous section are either already naturally present in foods, or produced by conventional processes such as cooking. Thus, unless the quantity of reaction products produced by irradiation is significantly greater than that ordinarily observed, they should be of little or no toxicological concern. In addition, there would be no toxicological concern should the fatty acid or amino acid content of a food be increased by radiation-induced decomposition of triglycerides or proteins.

Because of the lack of information on the absolute composition of irradiated and nonirradiated foods at $\mu g/kg$ and ng/kg levels, it is not known whether truly unique radiolytic products exist. It is possible that so-called unique products are also present in foods that have undergone conventional thermal processing. As it will be difficult to establish that such products exist, concern about their toxicological significance can only be speculative.

The United States Army's high-protein food-sterilization study has generated detailed analyses of 65 volatile chemicals in beef irradiated at 50 kGy

(Merritt, 1972; FASEB, 1979). Two of these were not radiolytic products, as irradiation had no effect on their concentrations. The remaining 63 chemicals formed a nearly homologous series of reaction products of triglycerides from the beef lipid fraction. In the conclusion of its report, a committee of the Federation of American Societies for Experimental Biology (FASEB, 1977) stated that "The Committee concluded that there were no grounds to suspect that the radiolytic compounds evaluated in this report would constitute any hazard to health to persons consuming reasonable quantities of beef irradiated in the described manner." The thermally sterilized control contained 23 of the 63 volatile chemicals; 40 therefore seemed to be unique to the irradiated lipid fraction. The FDA reported that only six of the 40 compounds could not be identified in volatile fractions of other nonirradiated foods (Food and Drug Administration, 1980). Of this subset of 63 volatile chemicals, therefore, only some 10% were considered unique by the FDA. The structures of the six chemicals were reported to be similar to molecules occurring in other food volatile fractions, and similar to those of some natural food constituents.

Re-examination by the current authors of the two studies referred to by the FDA in their 1980 report (Central Institute for Nutrition and Food Research, 1977; FASEB, 1977) revealed that only three of the 63 compounds (undecyne, pentadecadiene, and hexadecadiene) had not been found in nonirradiated foods. These three compounds, however, cannot be considered unusual. Though undecyne has not been reported in nonirradiated foods, decyne, containing one less carbon atom, is found in food. Similarly, pentadecadiene and hexadecadiene are each one carbon atom removed from tetradecadiene and heptadecadiene, both of which have been detected in nonirradiated foods. Because their very close homologues have been found, undecyne, pentadecadiene, and hexadecadiene in all probability exist at low levels in nonirradiated foods.

While the example cited above relates to a series of reaction products associated with a volatile fraction of irradiated food, there is no reason to believe that this is atypical. In other words, the example is likely to be typical of the relationship of nonvolatile radiolytic products and possibly unique radiolytic products both with one another and with radiolytic products that are constituents of other nonirradiated foods.

It might be naive to assume that there are no truly unique radiolytic products, which could be coupling products of radicals derived from lipids and proteins, resulting in dimers or cross-linked compounds. Enzymatic hydrolysis, though, would be expected to split most of these unique radiolytic products into common moieties such as fatty acids, amino acids, monosaccharides, and their reaction products resulting from the human digestive process.

Thermal decomposition of triglycerides, fatty acids, and fatty acid methyl esters produces a wide variety of n-alkanes, 1-alkenes, ketones, aldehydes, lactones, dimeric hydrocarbons and alcohols, together with carbon dioxide, carbon monoxide, hydrogen, dimer acids, and esters (Nawar, 1977). Comparisons have been made between these products and the typical radiolytic products formed in irradiated fats, and many similarities were noted. In addition, the dimeric compounds produced by heating methyl oleate were similar to those produced by the irradiation of potassium oleate.

It is quite reasonable to conclude, therefore, that unique radiolytic products, if indeed they exist, constitute an extremely small percentage of the total radiolytic products formed.

4.14 Summary and conclusions

No measurable radioactivity is induced in foods treated with ionizing radiation at internationally approved energy levels. The amount of ionizing radiation energy needed to produce the desired effects is generally far less than the amount of energy used in traditional methods of food processing such as cooking.

Over 30 years of research have shown that radiolytic products resulting from the treatment of foods with ionizing energy are very similar, if not identical, to those found in unprocessed foods or foods that have undergone conventional processing.

Concern about the production of compounds unique to the irradiation process is probably unfounded. Only the application of more sensitive analytical techniques, not yet available, to both irradiated and nonirradiated foodstuffs could establish whether they exist or not. Given the vast number of different types of food, such an undertaking would be unrealistic, and would produce results that were largely meaningless or even misleading.

Much has been learned about the chemistry of irradiated foods over the past three decades. The information has provided an important foundation for the assessment of the safety and nutritional adequacy of irradiated food.

References

Advisory Committee on Irradiated and Novel Foods (1986) *Report on the safety and wholesomeness of irradiated foods.* London, Her Majesty's Stationery Office.

Beyers M, Thomas AC (1979) Gamma-irradiation of sub-tropical fruits. 4. Changes in certain nutrients present in mangoes, papayas and litchis during canning, freezing and irradiation. *Journal of agricultural and food chemistry,* 27:48–51.

CAST (1986) *Ionizing energy in food processing and pest control. I. Wholesomeness of food treated with ionizing energy.* Ames, IA, Council for Agricultural Science and Technology (Report No. 109).

Central Institute for Nutrition and Food Research (1977) *Volatile compounds in foods*, 4th ed. Zeist.

Dauphin J, Saint-Lèbe LR (1977) Radiation chemistry of carbohydrates. In: Elias PS, Cohen AJ, eds. *Radiation chemistry of major food components*. Amsterdam, Elsevier, pp. 131–185.

Delincée H (1983) Recent advances in the radiation chemistry of proteins. In: Elias PS, Cohen AJ, eds. *Recent advances in food irradiation*, Amsterdam, Elsevier Biomedical, pp. 129–147.

Delincée H, Radola BJ (1974) Effect of gamma irradiation on the charge and size properties of horseradish peroxidase: individual isoenzymes. *Radiation research*, **59**:572–584.

Delincée H, Radola BJ (1975) Structural damage of gamma-irradiated ribonuclease revealed by thin-layer isoelectric focussing. *International journal of radiation biology*, **28**:565–579.

Diehl JF (1975) [Thiamine in irradiated foods. 1. Influence of various conditions and of time after irradiation.] *Zeitschrift für Lebensmittel-Untersuchung und-Forschung*, **157**:317–321 (In German).

Diehl JF (1979) [Reduction of radiation-induced vitamin losses by irradiation of foodstuffs at low temperature and by exclusion of atmospheric oxygen.] *Zeitschrift für Lebensmittel-Untersuchung und -Forschung*, **169**:276–280 (in German).

Diehl JF (1982) Radiolytic effects in foods. In: Josephson ES, Peterson MS, eds. *Preservation of foods by ionizing radiation*, Vol. 1. Boca Raton, FL, CRC Press, pp. 279–357.

Diehl JF (1990) *Safety of irradiated food*. New York, Marcel Dekker.

Diehl JF et al. (1979) Radiolysis of carbohydrates and of carbohydrate-containing foods. *Journal of agricultural and food chemistry*, **26**:15–20.

FAO (1984) *Codex General Standard for Irradiated Foods and Recommended International Code of Practice for the Operation of Radiation Facilities Used for the Treatment of Food*. Rome, Food and Agriculture Organization of the United Nations (CAC/Vol. XV-Ed.1).

FASEB (1977) *Evaluation of the health aspects of certain compounds found in irradiated beef*. Bethesda, MD, Life Sciences Research Office, Federation of American Societies for Experimental Biology.

FASEB (1979) *Evaluation of the health aspects of certain compounds found in irradiated beef*, supplements I and II. Bethesda, MD, Life Sciences Research Office, Federation of American Societies for Experimental Biology.

Food and Drug Administration (1980) *Recommendations for evaluating the safety of irradiated foods. Final report, July 1980.* Washington, DC.

Food and Drug Administration (1986) Irradiation in the production, processing, and handling of food. *Federal register*, **51**:13376–13399.

Galetto W et al. (1979) Irradiation treatment of onion powder: effects on chemical constituents. *Journal of food science*, **44**:591–595.

Green BE, Watts BM (1966) Lipid oxidation in irradiated cooked beef. *Food technology*, **20**(8):111–114.

Jensen M (1960) *Irradiation of berry fruit with reference to their industrial utilization.* Roskilde, Danish Atomic Energy Commission (Risö Report 16:77).

Kavalam JP, Nawar WW (1969) Effects of ionizing radiation on some vegetable fats. *Journal of the American Oil Chemists Society*, **46**:387–390.

Kennedy TS, Ley FJ (1971) Studies on the combined effect of gamma radiation and cooking on the nutritional value of food. *Journal of the science of food and agriculture*, **22**:146–148.

Liebster J, Kopoldova J (1964) The radiation chemistry of amino acids. *Advances in radiation biology*, **1**:157–226.

Merritt C Jr (1972) Qualitative and quantitative aspects of trace volatile components in irradiated foods and food substances. *Radiation research reviews*, **3**:353–368.

Merritt C Jr, Taub IA (1983) Commonality and predictability of irradiated products in irradiated meats. In: Elias PS, Cohen AJ, eds. *Recent advances in food irradiation.* Amsterdam, Elsevier Biomedical, pp. 27–57.

Moshonas MG, Shaw PE (1984) Effects of low-dose gamma irradiation on grapefruit products. *Journal of agricultural and food chemistry*, **32**:1098–1101.

Nagay NY, Moy JH (1985) Quality of gamma irradiated California Valencia oranges. *Journal of food science*, **50**:215–219.

Nawar WW (1977) Radiation chemistry of lipids. In: Elias PS, Cohen AJ, eds. *Radiation chemistry of major food components.* Amsterdam, Elsevier, pp. 21–61.

Nawar WW (1983) Radiolysis of nonaqueous components of foods. In: Josephson ES, Peterson MS, eds. *Preservation of food by ionizing radiation*, Vol. 2. Boca Raton, FL, CRC Press, pp. 75–124.

Nawar WW (1986) Volatiles from food irradiation. *Food reviews international*, **2**:45–78.

Proctor BE et al. (1952) Biochemical prevention of flavor and chemical changes in foods and tissues sterilized by ionizing radiation. *Food technology*, 6:237–242.

Proctor BE, O'Meara JP (1951) Effect of high-voltage cathode rays on ascorbic acid—*in vitro* and *in situ* experiments. *Industrial and engineering chemistry*, 43:718–721.

Radola BJ (1974) Identification of irradiated meat by thin layer gel chromatography and thin layer isoelectric focussing. In: *Identification of irradiated foodstuffs*. Luxembourg, Commission of the European Communities, pp. 27–43 (EUR 5126).

Romani RJ et al. (1963) Radiation physiology of fruit—ascorbic acid, sulphydryl and soluble nitrogen content of irradiated citrus. *Radiation botany*, 3:363–369.

Simic MG (1983) Radiation chemistry of water soluble food components. In: Josephson ES, Peterson MS, eds. *Preservation of food by ionizing radiation*, Vol. 2. Boca Raton, FL, CRC Press, pp. 1–73.

Sreenivasan A (1974) Compositional and quality changes in some irradiated foods. In: *Improvement of food quality by irradiation*. Vienna, International Atomic Energy Agency, pp. 129–155.

Taub IA (1983) Reaction mechanisms, irradiation parameters, and product formation. In: Josephson ES, Peterson MS, eds. *Preservation of food by ionizing radiation*, Vol. 2. Boca Raton, FL, CRC Press, pp. 125–166.

Terry AJ, McColl NP (1992) *Radiological consequences of food irradiation*. London, National Radiological Protection Board.

Thomas MH et al. (1981) EFfect of radiation and conventional processing on thiamin content of pork. *Journal of food science*, 46:824–828.

Thomas P, Dharkar SD, Sreenivasan A (1971) Effect of gamma irradiation on the post harvest physiology of five banana varieties grown in India. *Journal of food science*, 36:243–247.

Underdal B et al. (1973) The effect of ionizing radiation on the nutritional value of fish (cod) protein. *Lebensmittelwissenschaft und Technologie*, 6:90–93.

Urbain WM (1977) Radiation chemistry of proteins. In: Elias PS, Cohen AJ, eds. *Radiation chemistry of major food components*. Amsterdam, Elsevier, pp. 63–130.

Uzunov G et al. (1972) Changes in the soluble muscle proteins and isoenzymes of lactate dehydrogenase in irradiated beef meat. *International journal of radiation biology*, 22:437–442.

Vajdi M, Merritt C Jr (1985) Identification of adduct radiolysis products from pork fat. *Journal of the American Oil Chemists Society*, **62**:1252–1260.

von Sonntag C (1980) Free-radical reactions of carbohydrates as studied by radiation techniques. *Advances in carbohydrate chemistry and biochemistry*, **37**: 7–77.

WHO (1965) *The technical basis for legislation on irradiated food: report of a Joint FAO/IAEA/WHO Expert Committee.* Geneva, World Health Organization (WHO Technical Report Series, No. 316).

WHO (1981) *Wholesomeness of irradiated food: report of a Joint FAO/IAEA/WHO Expert Committee.* Geneva, World Health Organization (WHO Technical Report Series, No. 659).

Wills PA (1965) Some effects of gamma radiation on several varieties of Tasmanian potatoes. 2. Biochemical changes. *Australian journal of experimental agriculture and animal husbandry*, **5**:289–295.

Zegota H (1988) Suitability of Dukat strawberries for studying effects on shelf life of irradiation combined with cold storage. *Zeitschrift für Lebensmittel-Untersuchung und -Forschung*, **187**:111–114.

5.
Post-irradiation detection methods

5.1 Introduction

Early attempts to develop analytical techniques to determine whether foods have been subjected to ionizing radiation were concerned primarily with qualitative aspects, but more recently attention has also turned to the measurement of the absorbed dose.

Although much progress has been made, it is unlikely that rapid, routine analytical methods suitable for use in the enforcement of legislation on food irradiation will be available in the near future for all foods. To a large extent, enforcement will necessarily be based primarily on inspection of in-plant records (or other on-site monitoring). For imported foods, such in-plant inspection or control will rarely, if ever, be possible. It is expected, however, that foods that have been irradiated will be labelled to that effect by the exporting country. Post-irradiation detection methods provide the only means of controlling illegal imports of unlabelled irradiated products.

The analytical problem is complicated by the fact that most, if not all, of the chemicals formed as a result of irradiation are not unique to the irradiation process, e.g. they may be present naturally or produced by other food-treatment processes, such as thermal processing. Development of a universal method of detection has been hampered by this fact, and distinguishing irradiated from nonirradiated foods poses a formidable problem.

Much research has been carried out in the attempt to find methods for detecting whether food has been irradiated. Comprehensive reviews of the literature on such methods are contained in two recent publications (Sanderson, 1990; Delincée, 1991a). A shorter and more recent review is that of Stevenson (1992).

Methods of detecting irradiated foods should satisfy a number of criteria. The "perfect" method would be simple, inexpensive, rapid, reliable, use readily available instrumentation, require reasonably small sample sizes, allow for the detection of a wide range of absorbed doses, and not give false positives. In addition, it should preferably be of general application, measure the total absorbed dose, and be able to identify irradiated constituents in combination foods.

Most of the above requirements will probably not be met for some time. Current analytical techniques and those that seem likely to become available in the near future are not such as to permit the quantitative determination of absorbed dose. In addition, the method used will almost certainly vary by food type, so that a number of different tests will be required. International protocols exist for the testing and adoption of standardized analytical methods (IUPAC, 1990). Detection methods in accordance with these protocols will help to promote the acceptance of irradiated foods by governments, in commerce and, most importantly, by the consuming public.

5.2 International activities

Over the past 25 years or so, the subject of the detection of irradiated foods has been discussed at numerous meetings and symposia. Of these, only three of the larger international meetings have focused on detection methods.

The Commission of the European Communities organized conferences in 1970 (Luxembourg) and 1973 (Karlsruhe), but it was not until 1986 that the WHO Regional Office for Europe organized an international conference at Neuherberg, Germany, at which a WHO Working Group (Bögl et al., 1988) summarized the knowledge available at that time on analytical methods for identifying irradiated foods. The conclusion reached was that no universal method for detecting irradiated foods existed, but that methods were available for selected food types. However, most of the methods were in the early stages of development and few had the potential to measure the absorbed dose. However, the Working Group predicted that significant advances would be made in the near future, based on a number of new approaches outlined at the meeting.

Several countries have national programmes for developing detection methods, and coordinated efforts for that purpose are increasing; they include the recent establishment of a coordinated research programme by the Joint FAO/IAEA Division of Nuclear Techniques in Food and Agriculture. This is known as ADMIT (Analytical Detection Methods for Irradiation Treatment of Foods), involves 23 collaborating institutes, and is engaged in the study of analytical methods for a number of foods. Two collaborative activities on the use of electron spin resonance (ESR) and thermoluminescence (TL) techniques were initiated in 1990 by the Community Bureau of Reference of the Commission of the European Communities (BCR) and two workshops on new methods of detection were held in Cadarache, France, and in Ancona, Italy.

The first ADMIT meeting was held in Warsaw, Poland, in June 1990 (ADMIT, 1990). Convened by IAEA, it reviewed programme work and planned future research. Ladomery (1991) has outlined the analytical research currently under way in the ADMIT research programme. The type of food substrate, the food items under study, and the principle of the methods are summarized in Table 2. As can be seen, a wide variety of approaches are under investigation.

At the Warsaw meeting, it was reported that protocols for method validation had been developed by IUPAC jointly with the Association of Official Analytical Chemists (AOAC) and the International Organization for Standardization (ISO), in collaboration with the Codex Committee on Methods of Analysis and Sampling (IUPAC, 1990). It was concluded that international interlaboratory testing and validation were essential and proposed that ADMIT should organize and coordinate the work. Specialized research groups covering ESR, chemiluminescence (CL), TL, chemical methods, physical methods, and biological methods were established; they will exchange information, arrange collaborative studies and maintain close contact with the appropriate BCR subgroups. Delincée (1991a) reported that several methods would be ready for international collaborative study in 1992; these are listed in Table 3. Several interlaboratory collaborative trials have been carried out or are under way (ADMIT, 1992; Stevenson, 1992; Raffi et al., 1993).

5.3 Methods

Within the last 10 years, a number of investigators have reviewed the changes occurring in food after irradiation (Jeffries 1983; Chuaqui-Offermanns, 1987; Mitchell, 1987; Bradford, 1989; Hasselmann & Marchioni, 1989; Bögl, 1989, 1990; Grootveld & Jain, 1990; Delincée et al., 1988; Delincée & Ehlermann 1989). The changes may be chemical, physical, or biological each type having the potential to provide a means of detecting and measuring the effects of irradiation.

5.3.1 Chemical changes

The chemical changes brought about by the irradiation of foods result from the formation of free radicals by the reaction of ionizing radiation with food components, leading to a wide variety of radiolytic products. Free radicals are not produced solely by ionizing radiation, as they are also generated by many other processes, including heating, photolysis, catalysis by metal ions and enzymes, grinding, the use of ultrasound, and the reaction of food components with oxygen and peroxides. It is not surprising, therefore, that food irradiation produces chemical moieties already known to exist in foods.

In time, more radiolytic products are likely to be identified in non-irradiated foods. If unique radiolytic products were to be found, analytical detection methods could be based on them, and their presence would be proof that the foodstuff had been irradiated. It is now generally agreed that the likelihood of the existence of such compounds is extremely low. At one time o-tyrosine was thought to be a unique radiolytic product (Simic et al., 1983), but it has since been identified in several nonirradiated foods by Karam & Simic (1988a, b) and Hart et al. (1988). It has also been identified as

Table 2. Analytical research currently under way in the ADMIT research programme[a]

Substrate	Food	Technique
Food containing bones, shells, exoskeletons, inorganic matter	Spices, herbs, dry vegetables, poultry, meat, shellfish, fish, shrimp	Electron spin resonance
Food containing mineral particles, calcified cuticle, or shell	Spices, herbs, dry vegetables, shellfish	Thermoluminescence and chemiluminescence
Foods containing polymers, especially starch	Spices	Measurement of rheological changes (e.g. viscometry)
	Potatoes, dates, broad beans, wheat	Measurement of boiling point of aqueous extracts
Foods containing lipids	Poultry, meat, fish, spices	Lipid-derived volatile hydrocarbons Lipid-derived cyclobutanones
	Eggs, milk, nuts, soya flour	Lipid hyperoxidation
Foods containing protein	Chicken, pork, fish, shrimp	*o*-Tyrosine method
Foods containing DNA	Chicken, vegetables	Fragmentation of DNA measured by microelectrophoresis of single cells
Foods containing volatile substances	Spices	Measurement of chemical changes by gas-liquid chromatography
To be determined individually	Spices, herbs	Near-infrared spectrometry
Bulbous, aqueous vegetables (tubers, bulbs, roots)	Potatoes	Electrical impedance measurements
Foods containing seeds	Grapefruit, oranges, lemons	Inhibition by radiation of capacity of individual embryos to develop a shoot
Foods containing microorganisms	Spices, herbs	Combined use of DEFT and APC[b]

[a] From Ladomery (1991).
[b] DEFT: direct epifluorescent filter technique; APC: aerobic plate count.

Table 3. Methods ready for international collaborative study[a]

Substrate	Technique
Spices, herbs, dehydrated vegetables and other dry ingredients[b]	Thermoluminescence, chemiluminescence
Contaminant minerals in spices, grains, fruits and vegetables, bulbs and tubers[b]	Thermoluminescence
Chicken[b]	Electron spin resonance
Strawberries	Electron spin resonance
Chicken[b]	Lipid-derived volatiles
Potatoes	Electrical impedance
Chicken, seafood	o-Tyrosine method
Frozen seafood	DNA strand-breaks
Spices, herbs, dehydrated vegetables	Viscometry
Citrus and other fruits	Inhibition of seed germination

[a] From Delincée (1991a).
[b] Collaborative study being carried out (Delincée, 1993).

a product of the ultraviolet irradiation of aqueous solutions of phenylalanine by Hasselmann & Laustriat (1973).

Since irradiation of food involves the absorption of relatively small amounts of energy, chemical changes are less than those observed in the cooking process, where large amounts of energy are absorbed. Foods are complex mixtures of many substances, all of which compete with one another to absorb the ionizing radiation, so that the effects on any one component are expected to be minimal. This is in marked contrast to the effects of irradiation on pure chemicals in solution, where the impact is generally much greater. As it will be difficult to establish truly unique radiolytic products and the yields of the products that are formed are low, developing reliable analytical methods to measure chemical changes in irradiated foods continues to be a difficult task.

The measurement of relative amounts of particular chemicals selected on the basis of the food type is probably the most practical approach. Pattern recognition (or simplified versions of it) and analysis of variance have been applied to different foodstuffs in attempts to detect effects produced by irradiation.

Proteins

Changes in the chemical composition of proteins have been examined by a number of investigators using electrophoresis or gel permeation chromatography (Delincée et al. 1988) but with only limited success. The detection of protein-derived radiolytic products seems to offer some hope of success. Products derived from aromatic amino acids deserve investigation, as they are highly radiation-sensitive. A radiolytic product of the aromatic amino acid phenylalanine has been investigated in depth, as described below.

Phenylalanine reacts to produce o-, m-, and p-tyrosine (o-, m-, and p-hydroxyphenylalanine) (Dizdaroglu & Simic, 1980; Simic & de Graaf, 1981; Dizdaroglu et al., 1983; Simic et al., 1983, 1985; Solar, 1985). The *ortho* and *meta* isomers were once thought to be absent in natural proteins (Simic & de Graaf, 1981; Simic et al., 1983) and could thus serve as markers of irradiation (Karam & Simic, 1988a, b; Meier et al., 1988, 1989, 1990). Since the *ortho* isomer is produced in largest quantity by irradiation, it has been extensively studied. Since the level of o-tyrosine increases linearly with dose, the method was originally thought to be extremely promising. However, recently o-tyrosine has also been found in non-irradiated products (Karam & Simic, 1988a, b; Hart et al., 1988; Meier et al., 1988, 1989, 1990), and it is therefore no longer considered to be a unique radiolytic product.

In summary, the value of o-tyrosine as a possible indicator of exposure to irradiation is open to question, and further research is needed.

Lipids

Many investigators have studied lipid reaction products (Nawar, 1983a, b, 1986; Merritt & Taub, 1983; Merritt, 1984; Merritt et al., 1985; Vajdi & Merritt, 1985; Delincée, 1983). The studies have demonstrated that a relationship exists between the radiolytic products formed, lipid type and dosage. Attention has been focused on the volatile products, as these may be responsible for the off-flavours developed in irradiated meats. The main types of compounds found are hydrocarbons, aldehydes, ketones, methyl and ethyl esters, and free fatty acids. Cleavage of lipids occurs primarily near the ester carbonyl, producing alkanes and alkenes with 1 or 2 fewer carbon atoms.

Nawar & Balboni (1970) found that irradiation of pork gives rise to six major hydrocarbons whose concentrations increase linearly with dose. Nawar (1988) has proposed analysis for the volatile products as an indicator of irradiation, although he also found (Nawar, 1983a, 1988) that these chemicals are formed by autoxidation or heating. While the same volatile products are formed, the distribution patterns of individual products vary. Hydrocarbons with one or two fewer carbon atoms and aldehydes were judged to be most suitable as possible indicators of irradiation.

This simple approach to post-irradiation dosimetry appears highly promising and is currently under active investigation. Using a combination of high-pressure liquid chromatography and gas-liquid chromatography (GLC), Meier et al. (1990) found hydrocarbons and aldehydes in irradiated chicken flesh. Morehouse & Ku (1990) used a GLC method to identify irradiated frog legs; a good correlation between radiation dose and the resulting radiolytic products was observed. The authors also used the GLC procedure to estimate the applied dose in shrimp (Morehouse & Ku, 1992). Because the quantities being measured are extremely small (1–30 ng/kg), they cautioned that care had to be taken to avoid contamination, as several interfering hydrocarbons have been observed in both reagent blanks and nonirradiated shrimp; such contamination could possibly lead to misidentification of untreated shrimp as irradiated. The authors also reported that it was possible to improve the estimation of the absorbed dose by re-irradiation of the sample at several known absorbed doses and extrapolation of the results back to zero (method of standard addition). This technique has also been used by Desrosiers (1989) for the estimation of absorbed doses in shellfish by ESR. A German group (Bögl et al., 1993) has recently submitted the results of a collaborative trial, involving the determination of lipid volatiles, to the AOAC for publication and possible adoption as an AOAC method.

Other investigators reported encouraging results at the 1990 BCR workshop in Cadarache (Meier, 1991; Bögl, 1991; Raffi, 1991; Stevenson, 1991; Tuominen, 1991), since which several collaborative studies have been carried out (Delincée, 1993).

Cyclobutanones are also produced from fatty acids on irradiation, and offer an additional promising option for identification of irradiated foods (Stevenson, 1992).

Determination of lipid oxidation products is another possible approach, but has so far shown little promise as a means of identifying irradiated foods because such products can also be generated by a wide variety of conditions and factors, including storage, and exposure to oxygen, heat, trace metals, and enzymes.

In summary, the relatively simple measurement of lipid-derived volatile products is an approach of great potential, and is probably applicable to any food containing lipids, especially high-fat foods such as meat, fish, shellfish, and eggs. It has the distinct advantage as compared with other methods of requiring only expertise and equipment commonly available in most laboratories.

Carbohydrates

Carbohydrates react with ionizing radiation to produce mainly acids and carbonyl compounds (Dauphin & Saint-Lèbe, 1977; Adam, 1982; von Sonntag, 1987). Several investigators have studied the detection of carbonyl compounds, such as malonaldehyde, as an indicator of irradiation; these studies have been reviewed by Jeffries (1983) and by Delincée et al. (1988). However, attempts to use malonaldehyde as a marker chemical were largely unsuccessful for a number of reasons. Differences in, e.g. fruit variety, degree of ripening, storage and growth conditions, were found to cause greater variation in malonaldehyde levels than that produced by irradiation.

Physical rather than chemical changes in carbohydrates seem to hold more promise as a means of detection. Polysaccharides may be broken down by irradiation, resulting in a reduction in viscosity, an effect that will be discussed later.

In summary, given the present state of the art, chemical changes in carbohydrates do not appear promising as a means of identifying irradiated foods.

Nucleic acids

DNA is a component of most foods and is particularly sensitive to ionizing radiation. Gibbs & Wilkinson (1985) have thoroughly reviewed the area, as has Delincée (1991b). Radiation-induced changes in DNA have been described by von Sonntag (1987). Base damage, single-strand and double-strand breaks, and cross-linking between bases are the main effects on DNA.

Density-gradient centrifugation, alkaline elution techniques, HPLC, or alkaline gel electrophoresis may be used to detect strand breaks. Gibbs & Wilkinson (1985) have also suggested that enzymatic methods and electron microscopy could be used to detect DNA lesions. These approaches will be difficult to perfect because of the low concentrations of DNA in food.

To overcome this difficulty, immunological approaches might perhaps be employed (Parsons, 1987; Delincée et al., 1988; Swallow, 1988). Fuciarelli et al. (1985) have used an enzyme-linked immunosorbent assay (ELISA) to detect a radiolytic product in a nucleic acid solution, thereby demonstrating the potential of such an approach.

A number of investigators have examined the suitability of measuring thymine glycol as a means of identifying irradiated food (Swallow, 1988; Pfeilsticker & Lucas, 1987; Jabir et al., 1989; Deeble, 1990; von Sonntag, 1988). Although oxidation of thymine to thymine glycol can be demonstrated by fluorometry when solutions of thymine are irradiated, the attempts to verify this reaction in foods of complex composition, such as meat, have not shown promising results.

Strand breaks in DNA have also been investigated by several authors (Oestling & van Hofsten, 1988; Altmann et al., 1974; Swallow, 1988; Flegeau et al., 1988; Copin & Bourgeois, 1988, 1991a; Hasselmann & Marchioni, 1989, 1991; Spano, 1991; Deeble, 1991). However, it is known that food processing (e.g. cooking) also degrades DNA, so that the effects of irradiation are not specific.

A collaborative trial is under way using DNA fragmentation under the FAO/IAEA Cooperative Research Programme.

In summary, the evidence available is inadequate to demonstrate that changes in DNA can serve as a reliable indicator of irradiation. None the less, rapid developments in this field have produced some promising results (Stevenson, 1992).

Vitamins

Little work has been done on the identification of the radiolytic products of vitamins; for the most part, only the degree of degradation of the vitamins themselves has been measured. Because vitamins are present in very low concentrations, the detection and identification of the decomposition products will obviously be difficult.

Thayer (1988) investigated the use of thiamine as a possible marker of irradiation since an atypically low concentration might indicate exposure to ionizing radiation. This approach could not be used, however, if the food had undergone thermal processing such as cooking, as that would also result in loss of thiamine.

Spices

The measurement of changes in the volatile content of spices is an obvious method of detecting irradiation. Swallow (1988) suggested that the gas chromatographic pattern of spice volatiles should be examined since the appearance of new peaks might indicate exposure to radiation. Hasselmann et al. (1986) described the disappearance of a peak from black pepper, but Sjöberg et al. (1990b) failed to detect any differences between the treated and the untreated spice. Overall, differences in the patterns of volatiles from irradiated and nonirradiated spices appear to be small. In addition, the patterns of different varieties and batches of the same spice may differ significantly.

Hydrogen

Hydrogen is known to be produced by irradiation (Swallow, 1988) but, unless the gas is trapped in a food package such as a can, it will quickly diffuse out of the food. There are some indications, however, that the irradiation of pepper can be detected by measurement of ambient hydrogen. Dohmaru et al. (1989) reported that GLC analysis of the gas evolved after grinding irradiated pepper in a gas-tight ceramic mill indicated that hydrogen was liberated, and that treated pepper could be identified in this manner for 2–4 months, depending on storage temperature.

Other chemical changes

Liquor is irradiated in China to remove bitter components. Irradiation of ethanol itself produces three optical isomers of 2,3-butanediol, the $(+)$, $(-)$, and *meso* forms. No butanediol is found in nonirradiated liquors, and only the $(-)$ and *meso* forms may be produced by microbial action. Qi et al. (1990) reported that detection of $(+)$-2,3-butanediol was evidence of irradiation and that quantification of this substance enabled the absorbed dose to be estimated.

5.3.2 Physical properties

The physical properties of foods are sometimes altered on exposure to ionizing radiation. In particular, there may be damage to cell membranes, and measuring the effects of such damage could provide a way of detecting irradiation. Several approaches have been investigated, including the measurement of electrical impedance, electric potential, and viscosity, and thermal and near-infrared analysis.

Electrical impedance

Ionizing radiation can change the electrical impedance of a food matrix. Measurement can be made at various frequencies by inserting an electrode into the food. Ehlermann (1972) measured changes in impedance in fish as a means of estimating radiation dose, but biological variations in the impedance of fish themselves were found to be far greater than the changes brought about by irradiation in the dose ranges of interest.

More recent investigations by Hayashi (1988) showed that measurement of impedance at 50 and 5 kHz could be used to identify irradiated potatoes: the ratio of the impedances at these two frequencies was shown to be dose-dependent, unaffected by storage or growth conditions, and little affected by the variety chosen. It was concluded that the absorbed dose could be estimated as long as 6 months after irradiation if the potato variety was known. Other potato varieties are being investigated to determine the practicality and suitability of this approach under the FAO/IAEA Cordinated Research Programme.

In summary, measurement of impedance is potentially of value in determining whether potatoes have been irradiated. Studies are needed to determine whether the technique is more widely applicable.

Viscosity

The viscosity of homogenates and suspensions may be changed by irradiation; the changes can be measured by means of a rotational viscometer. Shrimp homogenates (Rhee, 1969) showed significant changes on irradiation, but these were small relative to biological variability. Spices, herbs, and dry vegetables have been investigated by Mohr & Wichmann (1985), Farkas et al. (1987, 1989, 1990a,b), Heide et al. (1987a, 1988), Heide & Bögl (1988a, 1990), and Wichmann et al. (1990). No firm conclusions could be reached; although changes in viscosity were observed, they were inconsistent—there were some increases and some decreases. Even different varieties of the same spice behaved differently. Sample preparation may also significantly affect the results.

One encouraging aspect of this approach is that viscosity is relatively stable on storage, so that changes due to irradiation can be detected even after several years. Farkas et al. (1990a) suggested that viscosity changes in ground pepper could be used as a basis for a rapid, simple method for irradiated spices, but also showed that high humidity can lead to significant changes in the physical properties of spices.

Thermal analysis

Rustichelli (1991), using differential scanning calorimetry (DSC), recently observed differences between irradiated and nonirradiated chicken. DSC also detected differences in irradiated cod and mushrooms (Kent, 1991). Here again, the approach needs to be investigated more fully so as to elucidate the changes brought about by irradiation.

Near-infrared analysis

This method is based on the near-infrared reflectance characteristics of food. Suzuki et al. (1988) used the second derivative of the near-infrared (NIR) spectrum to distinguish irradiated from nonirradiated spices. Research in this area, however, is still in its very early stages.

Electron spin resonance

Exposure of foods to ionizing radiation generally produces free radicals (see Chapter 4) which may be determined by a variety of techniques, ESR being the method of choice for direct detection. Although ESR is a well established, nondestructive method of free radical analysis, the equipment is expensive and highly skilled operators are required. It was suggested several years ago that ESR could be used as a detection technique (e.g. Dodd et al., 1985; Delincée et al., 1988; Onderdelinden & Strackee, 1974), and it has indeed shown great promise. Its application to various types of food is discussed below.

Fruit

Strong ESR signals from strawberry achenes irradiated at 10 kGy were found by Dodd et al. (1985), but differentiation at low doses was difficult because similar signals were found from the nonirradiated fruit, which were believed to be similar to those from melanin-type pigments (Goodman et al., 1989). Raffi et al. (1988) found a signal unique to the achenes of irradiated strawberries, which increased with dose and was independent of the method of preparation, but decayed on storage. However, the test identified all samples irradiated at a dose of 1 kGy or more followed by 20 days of storage at 5°C, i.e. the expected shelf-life of fresh strawberries. The tests were conducted on seven varieties offered for sale in France; additional work is needed to determine whether the technique is applicable to other varieties, and whether it may be extended to other fruits.

Goodman et al. (1989) also used ESR with oranges, grapefruit, and grapes. The signals from the seeds of oranges and grapefruit were not significantly increased by irradiation, and decayed on storage, leading to the conclusion that the technique was of little value. Later, Stachowicz et al. (1992) reported relatively stable ESR signals from the seeds of irradiated oranges and grapefruit.

Goodman et al. (1989) found that a small spectral component from the seeds of irradiated grapes was absent in nonirradiated samples; this may be related to the radiation-specific signal reported by Raffi et al. (1988) from strawberries, raspberries, bilberries, and redcurrants. More recently, Raffi & Agnel (1989) reported that this signal was caused by a cellulose radical, thought to be present in all irradiated fruits. There may be interference from other radicals, as other researchers (Stachowicz et al., 1992) apparently did not find this specific signal. It was observed by Desrosiers & McLaughlin (1989) with mango seeds, but decayed quickly, and could not be found with most other fruits. These conflicting results indicate that careful study is necessary before firm conclusions can be drawn.

Bulbs
The ESR technique appears not to be suitable for bulbs, as the radiation-induced signal from the outer skins of onion, garlic, and shallot was also produced by the nonirradiated samples and decayed quickly (Desrosiers & McLaughlin, 1989).

Grains
ESR does not seem to be suitable for grains, since the signal fades on storage. Signals have been detected with barley exposed to doses as high as 10 kGy, but the effects of the lower commercially used doses have not been investigated (Raffi et al., 1987).

Meat
A number of investigators have studied ESR signals from the bones of irradiated meat, e.g. Dodd et al. (1985, 1988, 1989); Lea et al. (1988); Desrosiers & Simic (1988); Goodman et al. (1989); Stevenson & Gray (1989); Gray & Stevenson (1989a, b); Gray et al. (1990); Stachowicz et al. (1992); and Meier et al. (1990). A typical signal from bone is observed on the irradiation of pork, veal, beef, or chicken. While signals native to nonirradiated samples were found, they could easily be distinguished from those produced by irradiation.

The importance of sample preparation was pointed out by Stevenson & Gray (1989) and Gray & Stevenson (1989a, b). A linear relationship has been found between dose and ESR signal in the range 1–25 kGy, but at 25 kGy, the response curve reaches a plateau (Lea et al., 1988). Lea et al. (1988) obtained a detection limit for chicken of 50 Gy, while Dodd et al. (1989) and Desrosiers & Simic (1988) reported a limit of 100 Gy.

Older animals give rise to more intense ESR signals because their bones are more highly mineralized and crystalline (Stachowicz et al., 1992; Gray et al., 1990). More intense ESR signals are also obtained from compact than from spongy bones because of the difference in mineralization. ESR signals from irradiated chicken bone increased linearly with dose and the slope increased linearly with age (Gray et al., 1990), so that the age of the chicken must be taken into account if ESR is to be used for quantification of the absorbed dose. The signal from chicken bone is relatively stable in storage. The signal was also slightly reduced after cooking (Lea et al., 1988; Gray & Stevenson, 1989b).

Similar results have been obtained for other poultry types (Lea et al., 1988; Dodd et al., 1989), and frog legs have been investigated by Raffi et al. (1989), Morehouse & Ku (1990), Morehouse et al. (1991), and Dodd et al. (1989). Raffi et al. found that the ESR signal was proportional to the dose up to 14 kGy, and remained constant for 2 years. Mechanically deboned turkey meat was analysed by Gray & Stevenson (1989a) who measured the ESR signal in the bone fragments after digestion of the flesh. The radiation dose could be estimated using a nonirradiated sample as a control. The dose may also be measured by re-irradiation of the sample bone fragments (Dodd et al., 1988, 1989).

Delincée (1991a) urged that a large-scale collaborative study should be carried out to determine the suitability of ESR and pointed out that at least three collaborative trials (two organized by the United Kingdom Ministry of Agriculture, Fisheries and Food, and the third by the European Community Bureau of References) were under way. Some of the results have already been published (Stevenson, 1992).

Seafood
It is also possible to use ESR to detect radiation treatment of fish and shellfish because they contain calcified material. Fish bone produces a lower signal than pork bone (Dodd et al., 1988; Goodman et al., 1989), no doubt because of its lower crystallinity. On the other hand, mussel shell produces a very strong signal, about 300 times greater than that from fish bone and 1000 times greater than that from shrimp (Desrosiers, 1989). Desrosiers (1989) and Stachowicz et al. (1992) found that the ESR signal from fish bone increased linearly with dose, and that there was a relatively small decrease in the signal after several months.

Morehouse & Desrosiers (1993) and Morehouse & Ku (1992) found that the ESR spectrum of shrimp shell was more complex than originally reported, depended on how the shell was processed, and was species- and batch-dependent; however, it was possible to distinguish irradiated from non-irradiated shrimp in some cases. It was concluded that the detection of irradiated shrimp would have to be limited to samples that exhibited a characteristic, distinct ESR spectrum as compared with a nonirradiated control.

An ESR signal can be obtained from nonirradiated shrimp shell, but irradiation produces new peaks. Dodd et al. (1985), Desrosiers (1989) and Goodman et al. (1989) reported quite different ESR spectra, possibly indicating differences in shrimp variety, age, source, or the specific part of the exoskeleton sampled. The spectra are complex, so that it may be possible to use estimation of the absorbed dose as a means of distinguishing irradiated from nonirradiated shrimp. Further study is obviously necessary.

Dodd et al. (1989) estimated the radiation dose in mussel shell by re-irradiation and extrapolation of the signal to zero. Desrosiers (1989) reported that he was able to distinguish irradiated from nonirradiated shell, though the signal decayed with time.

Spices

Some investigators have reported that ESR signals from spices decay relatively rapidly (Delincée et al., 1988; Shieh & Wierbicki, 1985), though in some cases (Yang et al., 1987) signals from a number of spices could be detected after 34 days, and Morishita et al. (1988) were able to distinguish between irradiated and nonirradiated pepper for up to 13 weeks. It should be noted that storage periods of many months are not uncommon for spices.

Summary

As a qualitative tool, ESR has been shown to be effective for bone-containing foods and possibly also shellfish, and some fruits and spices. Several collaborative trials have been carried out (BCR, 1992). Quantitatively, the technique may be useful for bone, and further study is indicated.

Luminescence

Luminescence is the emission of light when trapped energy is liberated either by the addition of a chemical (chemiluminescence) or by heating (thermoluminescence), when trapped charge carriers are released. Luminescence techniques are the most thoroughly investigated of all the methods used to detect exposure to irradiation.

Chemiluminescence

In chemiluminescence (CL) studies, an alkaline luminol–haemin solution is added to the dry substance and the CL response measured with a light detector. Spices, herbs, and other dry ingredients have been studied extensively by the CL technique (Heide & Bögl, 1988a, 1990). A number of problems with the technique have become apparent including variation of the CL intensity from one spice to another and between different batches of the same spice, failure of the signal to increase with increasing dose for some spices, fading of the signal with time, poor reproducibility, and quenching of the signal by exposure to water vapour.

Because of these problems, nonirradiated controls would be highly desirable for comparative purposes, but will rarely be available for routine use. This technique will generally be successful, therefore, only in conjunction with others. For a number of products, however, identification appears to be successful (Heide & Bögl, 1988a, 1990); dehydrated juniper berries, carrots, mushrooms, cardamom, garlic, laurel, and celery are all commodities for which the CL technique may be used.

Luminescence detection methods have been the subject of two collaborative studies on irradiated spices: the first, in 1985 used CL (Heide et al., 1986a; Heide & Bögl, 1988b), while the second in 1988 used both CL and TL (Heide et al., 1989a,b). In the first, 63% of the samples were correctly classified, but a 93% success rate was achieved for commodities such as celery, coriander, turmeric (curcuma), and juniper berries, so that the technique showed great promise for certain selected spices.

About 65% of the irradiated samples were correctly identified in the second study, which involved 12 European investigators. Again, the results were very encouraging for certain of the commodities studied, including cardamom, carrots, garlic, coriander, mushrooms, juniper berries, and onions. These conclusions, however, are valid only for the specific samples examined as other lots may give different results.

Thermoluminescence

Thermoluminescence has been used for irradiation dosimetry (Mahesh & Vij, 1985), and Heide and co-workers have used it to identify a variety of irradiated foods (Heide & Bögl, 1984, 1987, 1988a, c, d, 1990; Heide et al., 1986b, 1987b). As with CL, the method is simple to use. The dry sample is heated at the rate of 10 °C per second to a temperature of 300–400 °C and the light emitted is measured. The samples are reheated to give a background value and the difference between the two values is used as a measure of the light emitted. Here again, the technique has been studied intensively; over 40 different commodities have been investigated.

A number of problems have emerged. Different spices, as well as batches of the same spice from different producers, varied greatly in their response (Heide et al., 1987b). Replicate measurements gave highly variable results and degradation of the signal with time has been observed (Moriarty et al., 1988). However, TL may be preferable to CL for certain spices. Heide & Bögl (1988a, 1990), for example, reported the successful use of TL for 20 spices. Very promising results using TL techniques were also obtained in the second collaborative trial mentioned above (Heide et al., 1989a, b). Of 495 samples examined, 99% were correctly classified, and no false positives were reported. For certain spices, then, the TL approach has great potential. It is also noteworthy that the Government of Germany uses a combination of CL and

TL for routine screening in its food inspection laboratories (Anon., 1989a, b, c, d).

Sanderson et al. (1989a,b) recently demonstrated that contaminating minerals in spices give rise to TL. This may explain why different batches of spices give different results. The use of TL for field crops, such as vegetables, fruits, and grains, is therefore possible, as they will all contain some minerals.

These results have been confirmed by Gökshu-Oegelmann & Regulla (1989) and Heide & Bögl (1989), who used TL for the identification of irradiated strawberries. Sanderson (1991) also described the use of photostimulated luminescence and the potential application of this technique to herbs, spices, bones, and shells. Sjöberg et al. (1990) reported that the use of thermoluminescence for detecting contaminating minerals is being investigated at the Technical Research Centre in Finland and at the University of Helsinki for purposes of import control.

Both CL and TL techniques appear to be suitable for the detection of certain irradiated foods, as demonstrated in several collaborative trials (Stevenson, 1992; Anon, 1993, 1993a).

5.3.3 Histological, morphological and biological effects

Histological and morphological effects

The cell structure of plant and animal tissue may be affected by ionizing radiation, and some of the changes may be observable macroscopically, so that they could serve as detectors of irradiation. Most of the procedures, however, take a long time to complete, often even weeks.

Sparenberg (1974) considered that tissue culture and detection of morphological changes in buds of irradiated potatoes were reliable indicators of irradiation. More recently, Kawamura et al. (1989a) reported that changes in the percentage germination of grapefruit seeds could be used to detect irradiation. Variety, harvest date, and storage did not seem to affect the results. The test, while simple to perform, requires 6–14 days to carry out, though it may be possible to reduce the time necessary by increasing the germination temperature and adding gibberellin. This method has also been used with other citrus fruits, such as oranges and lemons (Kawamura et al., 1989b) and could perhaps be extended to all seed-containing fruits.

More study is needed on a rapid rooting test for onions (Zehnder, 1984), a test for mushrooms (Zehnder, 1988), the visualization of enzyme activity in irradiated potatoes (Jona & Fronda, 1990), and the formation of hyphae after culturing small pieces of mushroom (Bugyaki & Heinemann, 1972). The embryo test of Kawamura et al. (1989a) holds promise for foods containing viable seeds, and further study of it is also indicated.

Microflora

Many foods are known to be contaminated with microorganisms. The direct epifluorescent filter technique (DEFT) and aerobic plate count (APC) can be used together to measure the total microorganisms present before and after irradiation. Foods may be judged to have been irradiated if the DEFT count is larger than the APC count by a factor of more than 10^4. Sjöberg et al. (1990) considered the combined use of DEFT and APC to be a suitable method for detecting the irradiation of foods, particularly spices. They also reported that the technique was being investigated by the Technical Research Centre in Finland and the University of Helsinki for use in the control of imports.

Betts et al. (1988) examined different meats irradiated with doses up to 25 kGy, with promising results. McWeeny et al. (1990) used a similar approach in developing a bacterial screening test.

Commodities such as strawberries and seafood have been investigated, but a number of problems have been identified. Kampelmacher (1988) reported that it might not be possible to obtain meaningful results for strawberries grown in greenhouses or on plastic sheets, as microbial counts will be very low. In addition, the doses used for disinfestation or for delaying ripening are lower than those used to preserve or pasteurize the fruit. The same holds true for seafood (van Spreekens & Toepoel, 1978; Kampelmacher, 1988), although the reduction in microbial load obviously leads to a shift in the microflora. Colin et al. (1989) also suggested the use of this technique for the identification of irradiated chicken.

The resistance to radiation of 30 microbial strains from irradiated and nonirradiated chicken and smoked salmon was studied by Copin & Bourgeois (1992). Differences in the samples could be detected by re-irradiation and subsequent counting. The results of a collaborative study organized by the BCR were published recently (Sjöberg, 1993).

5.4 Harmonization of protocols and testing strategies

There is an obvious need for those publishing the results of collaborative studies to use harmonized protocols. At times, methods have been poorly standardized; definitions of precision have often been presented in formats of little practical value to the user, and other critical performance characteristics (e.g. accuracy, limit of quantification, etc.) have been inadequately defined. The availability of sound, properly validated analytical methods that are in line with international recommendations, e.g. the IUPAC protocols on standard methods (IUPAC, 1990), will help to promote the acceptance of irradiated foods.

None of the methods described here have been internationally recognized, but within Europe a round robin test programme, initiated at the BCR meeting in Ancona, Italy, in 1991, is being developed (Leonardi et al., 1992). Generally speaking, the methods currently available can be divided into (*a*) screening methods, which can be used to indicate whether a food has been treated or not, (*b*) detection methods, which provide a certain degree of assurance of irradiation treatment, and (*c*) quantitative methods.

The screening methods of major interest include the direct epifluorescent filter technique/aerobic plate count test (DEFT/APC), as well as different methods based on electrophoresis which show that DNA has been damaged.

Detection methods that can be used to confirm the screening test results include TL, ESR, and the identification of volatiles such as alkanes and alkenes, and of alkylcyclobutanes.

5.5 Summary and conclusions

Rapid progress has been made over the past few years in the development of reliable analytical methods to detect whether food has been subjected to ionizing radiation. The methods currently under development range from the very simple, using readily available equipment and expertise, to sophisticated techniques calling for highly skilled scientists.

Many of these methods have been or are being tested in international collaborative studies (Table 3, p. 54). In Germany, both TL and CL are used for routine testing of spices, herbs, and dry ingredients.

No truly universal detection methods currently exist. Future studies, especially those on DNA, may some day result in approaches that will make universal methods a reality. Until such time as these methods are available, it may be necessary to rely on a battery of tests to detect the effects of irradiation on a variety of foods. There is also a clear need for readily available reference materials, the harmonization of testing protocols, and international collaborative testing.

References

Adam S (1982) Radiolysis of α,α'-trehalose in concentrated aqueous solution; the effect of co-irradiated proteins and lipids. *International journal of radiation biology*, **42**:531–544.

ADMIT (1990) *Co-ordinated Research Programme on Analytical Detection Methods for Irradiation Treatment of Foods. First Research Co-ordination Meeting, Warsaw (Jachranka), Poland, 25–29 June 1990*. Vienna, International Atomic Energy Agency.

ADMIT (1992) *Co-ordinated Research Programme on Analytical Detection Methods for Irradiation Treatment of Foods. Second Research Coordination Meeting, Budapest, Hungary, 15–19 June 1992*. Vienna, International Atomic Energy Agency.

Altmann H et al. (1974) Tests to identify irradiated meat. In: *The identification of irradiated foodstuffs. Proceedings of an international colloquium*. Luxembourg, Commission of the European Communities, pp. 61–65.

Anon (1989a) Untersuchung von Lebensmitteln. Nachweis einer Strahlenbehandlung (ionisierende Strahlen) bei Gewürzen durch Messung der Chemilumineszenz. [Testing of foodstuffs. Detection of irradiation (ionizing radiation) of spices by measurement of chemiluminescence.] In: *Amtl. Sammlung Untersuch. Verfahren* nach 35 LMBG, L26.00–2, L53.00–3. Berlin, Beuth Verlag.

Anon (1989b) Untersuchung von Lebensmitteln. Nachweis einer Strahlenbehandlung (ionisierende Strahlen) bei Gemüseerzeugnissen (Trackengemüse) durch Messung der Chemilumineszenz. [Testing of foodstuffs. Detection of irradiation (ionizing radiation) of vegetable products (dried vegetables) by measurement of chemiluminescence.] In: *Amtl. Sammlung Untersuch. Verfahren* nach 35 LMBG, L53.00–2, L26.00–3. Berlin, Beuth Verlag.

Anon (1989c) Untersuchung von Lebensmitteln. Nachweis einer Strahlenbehandlung (ionisierende Strahlen) bei Gewürzen durch Messung der Thermolumineszenz. [Testing of foodstuffs. Detection of irradiation (ionizing radiation) of spices by measurement of thermoluminescence.] In: *Amtl. Sammlung Untersuch. Verfahren* nach 35 LMBG, L53.00–2. Berlin, Beuth Verlag.

Anon (1989d) Untersuchung von Lebensmitteln. Nachweis einer Strahlenbehandlung (ionisierende Strahlen) bei Gemüseerzeugnissen (Trockengemüse) durch Messung der Thermolumineszenz. [Testing of foodstuffs. Detection of irradiation (ionizing radiation) of vegetable products (dried vegetables) by measurement of thermoluminescence.] In: *Amtl. Sammlung Untersuch. Verfahren* nach 35 LMBG, L26.00–2. Berlin, Beuth Verlag.

Anon (1993) Thermoluminescence analysis to detect irradiated spice and herb mixtures: an intercomparison study. *Sozep hefte*, 2/1993.

Anon (1993a) Thermoluminescence analysis to detect irradiated fruit and vegetables: an intercomparison study. *Sozep hefte*, 3/1993.

BCR (1992) *BCR information, chemical analysis, electron spin resonance: intercomparison studies on irradiated foodstuffs*. Brussels (EUR 13630).

Betts RP (1988) The detection of irradiated foods using the direct epifluorescent filter technique. *Journal of applied bacteriology*, **64**: 329–335.

Bögl KW (1989) Identification of irradiated foods—methods, developments and concepts. *International journal of applied radiation and isotopes*, **40**: 1203.

Bögl KW (1990) Methods for identification of irradiated food. *Radiation physics and chemistry*, **35**: 301–310.

Bögl KW (1991) Activities of the German Federal Health Office in the field on detection of irradiated food. In: Raffi JJ, Belliardo JJ, eds. *Potential new methods of detection of irradiated food.* Luxembourg, Commission of the European Communities (BCR Workshop, EUR-13331).

Bögl KW et al., eds. (1988) *Health impact, identification, and dosimetry of irradiated foods. Report of a WHO Working Group.* Neuherberg, Institut für Strahlenhygiene des Bundesgesundheitsamtes (ISH-125).

Bögl KW et al. (1993) Gas chromatographic analysis of volatile hydrocarbons to detect irradiated chicken, pork and beef: an intercomparison method. *Sozep hefte*, 1/1993.

Bradford WR (1989) Aspects of implementation of food irradiation and identification of irradiated products. *Food irradiation newsletter*, **13**:55–57.

Bugyaki L, Heinemann P (1972) Identification des champignons irradiés. *Atomkernenergie*, **19**:261.

Chuaqui-Offermanns N (1987) *The identification of irradiated fish: a review.* Atomic Energy of Canada (AECL-9095).

Colin P et al. (1989) Etude des possibilités de différenciation par la voie microbiologique des volailles et produits transformés ayant subi ou non un traitement ionisant. *Viandes et produits carnés*, **10**:17–19.

Copin MP, Bourgeois C (1988) Détection des produits alimentaires ionisés. *Bretagne agro alimentaire*, **15**:2.

Copin MP, Bourgeois C (1991a) Development of a DNA filtration method. In: Raffi JJ, Belliardo JJ, eds. *Potential new methods of detection of irradiated food.* Luxembourg, Commission of the European Communities (BCR Workshop, EUR-13331), pp. 22–26.

Copin MP, Bourgeois C (1991b) Determination of the radioresistance of the microbial strains remaining on the product. In: Raffi JJ, Belliardo JJ, eds. *Potential new methods of detection of irradiated food.* Luxembourg, Commission of the European Communities (BCR Workshop, EUR-13331), pp. 91–99.

Copin MP, Bourgeois C (1992) Application of microbiological methods to detect irradiated poultry products. In: Leonardi M, Raffi JJ, Belliardo JJ, eds, *Recent advances on detection of irradiated food.* Luxembourg, Commission of the European Communities (BCR Workshop, EUR-14315), pp. 78–88.

Dauphin J.-F, Saint-Lèbe L (1977) Radiation chemistry of carbohydrates. In: Elias PS, Cohen AJ, eds. *Radiation chemistry of major food components.* Amsterdam, Elsevier, pp. 131–185.

Deeble DJ (1991) The detection of irradiated food based on modification to DNA. In: Raffi JJ, Belliardo JJ, eds. *Potential new methods of detection of irradiated food.* Luxembourg, Commission of the European Communities (BCR Workshop, EUR-13331).

Delincée H (1983) Recent advances in radiation chemistry of lipids. In: Elias PS, Cohen AJ, eds. *Recent advances in food irradiation*, Amsterdam, Elsevier Biomedical, p. 89.

Delincée H (1991a) *Analytical detection methods for irradiated foods: a review of the current literature.* Vienna, International Atomic Energy Agency (TEC-DOC-587).

Delincée H (1991b) Introduction to DNA methods. In: Raffi JJ, Belliardo JJ, eds. *Potential new methods of detection of irradiated food.* Luxembourg, Commission of the European Communities (BCR Workshop, EUR 13331), p. 5.

Delincée H (1993) Control of irradiated food. Recent developments in analytical detection methods. *Radiation physics and chemistry,* 42:351–357.

Delincée H, Ehlermann DAE (1989) Recent advances in the identification of irradiated food. *Radiation physics and chemistry,* 34:877–890.

Delincée H et al. (1988) The feasibility of an identification of radiation processed food. In: Bögl KW et al., eds. *Health impact identification and dosimetry of irradiated foods. Report of a WHO Working Group.* Neuherberg, Institut für Strahlenhygiene des Bundesgesundheitsamtes (ISH–125), p. 58.

Desrosiers MF (1989) Gamma-irradiated seafoods: identification and dosimetry by electron paramagnetic resonance spectroscopy. *Journal of agricultural and food chemistry,* 37:96.

Desrosiers MF, McLaughlin WL (1989) Examination of gamma irradiated fruits and vegetables by electron spin resonance spectroscopy. *Radiation physics and chemistry,* 34:895–898.

Desrosiers MF, Simic MG (1988) Postirradiation dosimetry of meat by electron spin resonance of bones. *Journal of agricultural and food chemistry,* 36:601.

Dizdaroglu MG, Simic MG (1980) Radiation induced conversion of phenylalanine to tyrosine. *Radiation research,* 83:437.

Dizdaroglu MG et al. (1983) Identification of some OH radical-induced products of lysozyme. *International journal of radiation biology,* 43:185.

Dodd NJF et al. (1985) Use of ESR to identify irradiated food. *Radiation physics and chemistry,* 26:451–453.

Dodd NJF et al. (1988) ESR detection of irradiated food. *Nature,* 334:387.

Dodd NJF et al. (1989) The ESR detection of irradiated food. *International journal of applied radiation and isotopes,* 40:1211.

Dohmaru M et al. (1989) Identification of irradiated pepper with the level of hydrogen gas as a probe. *Radiation research,* 120:552.

Ehlermann D (1972) The possible identification of an irradiation treatment of fish by means of electrical (ac) resistance measurement. *Journal of food science*, **37**:501.

Farkas J et al. (1987) Preliminary studies on the feasibility of an identification of some irradiated dry ingredients by viscosimetric measurements. In: *Proceedings of the XVIIIth Annual Meeting of the European Society of Nuclear Methods in Agriculture, 30 August–4 September 1987, Stara Zagora, Bulgaria.*

Farkas J et al. (1989) Further experiments on the detection of irradiation of dry food ingredients based on starch degradation. *Radiation physics and chemistry*, **34**:1027.

Farkas J et al. (1990a) Identification of irradiated dry ingredients on the basis of starch damage. *Radiation physics and chemistry*, **35**:324–328.

Farkas J et al. (1990b) Detection of some irradiated spices on the basis of radiation induced damage of starch. *Radiation physics and chemistry*, **36**:621–627.

Flegeau J et al. (1988) Detection of irradiated Norway lobsters by DNA elution method. In: Bögl KW et al., eds. *Health impact, identification, and dosimetry of irradiated foods. Report of a WHO Working Group.* Neuherberg, Institut für Strahlenhygiene des Bundesgesundheitsamtes (ISH-125), pp. 453–460.

Fuciarelli AF et al. (1985) An immunochemical probe for 8,5′-cycloadenosine-5′-monophosphate and its deoxy analog in irradiated nucleic acids. *Radiation research*, **104**:272.

Gibbs PA, Wilkinson VM (1985) *Feasibility of detecting irradiated foods by reference to the endogenous microflora: a literature review.* Leatherhead, Food Research Association (Scientific and Technical Survey, No. 149).

Gökshu-Oegelmann HY, Regulla DF (1989) Detection of irradiated food. *Nature*, **340**:23.

Goodman BA et al. (1989) Electron spin resonance spectroscopy of some irradiated foodstuffs. *Journal of the science of food and agriculture*, **47**:101–111.

Gray R, Stevenson MH (1989a) Detection of irradiated deboned turkey meat using electron spin resonance spectroscopy. *Radiation physics and chemistry*, **34**:899–902.

Gray R, Stevenson MH (1989b) The effect of post-irradiation cooking on the ESR signal in irradiated chicken drumsticks. *International journal of food science and technology*, **24**:447–450.

Gray R et al. (1990) The effect of irradiation dose and age of bird on the ESR signal in irradiated chicken drumsticks. *Radiation physics and chemistry*, **35**:284–287.

Grootveld M, Jain R (1990) Recent advances in the development of a diagnostic test for irradiated foodstuffs. *Free radical research communications*, **6**:271–292.

Hart RJ et al. (1988) Technical note: occurrence of *o*-tyrosine in non-irradiated foods. *International journal of food science and technology*, **23**: 643.

Hasselmann C, Laustriat G (1973) Photochimie des acides amines aromatiques en solution. I. DL-Phenylalanine, DL-tyrosine et L-dopa. *Photochemistry and photobiology*, **17**:275.

Hasselmann C, Marchioni E (1989) La détection des aliments ionisés. *Annales des falsifications de l'expertise chimique et toxicologique*, **82**:169.

Hasselmann C, Marchioni E (1991) Studies of mitochondrial DNA for detection of irradiated meat. In: Raffi JJ, Belliardo JJ, eds. *Potential new methods of detection of irradiated food*, Luxembourg, Commission of the European Communities (BCR Workshop, EUR-13331).

Hasselmann C et al. (1986) Mise en évidence de l'irradiation des aliments par des méthodes physico-chimiques. *Medecine et nutrition*, **22**:121–126.

Hayashi T (1988) Identification of irradiated potatoes by impedemetric methods. In: Bögl KW et al., eds. *Health impact, identification, and dosimetry of irradiated foods. Report of a WHO Working Group*. Neuherberg, Institut für Strahlenhygiene des Bundesgesundheitsamtes (ISH-125), pp. 432–452.

Hegi ME et al. (1989) Detection by ^{32}P postlabeling of thymidine glycol in gamma-irradiated DNA. *Carcinogenesis*, **10**:43.

Heide L, Bögl W (1984) *Die Messung der Thermolumineszenz—ein neues Verfahren zur Identifizierung strahlenbehandelter Gewürze*. [Measurement of thermoluminescence—a new method of identifying irradiated spices]. Neuherberg, Institut für Strahlenhygiene des Bundesgesundheitsamtes (ISH-58).

Heide L, Bögl W (1987) Identification of irradiated spices with thermo- and chemiluminescence measurements. *International journal of food science and technology*, **22**:93–103.

Heide L, Bögl KW (1988a) Fortschritte bei der Identifizierung bestrahlter Gewürze durch Messung der Chemilumineszenz, Thermolumineszenz und Viskosität. [Progress in the identification of irradiated spices by measurement of chemiluminescence, thermoluminescence and viscosity]. *Fleischwirtschaft*, **68**: 1559–1564.

Heide L, Bögl W (1988b) Routine application of luminescence techniques to identify irradiated spices—a first countercheck trial with 7 different research and food control laboratories. In: Bögl KW et al., eds. *Health impact, identification, and dosimetry of irradiated foods. Report of a WHO Working Group*. Neuherberg, Institut für Strahlenhygiene des Bundesgesundheitsamtes (ISH-125), pp. 233–244.

Heide L, Bögl W (1988c) Thermoluminescence and chemiluminescence investigations of irradiated food—a general survey. In: Bögl KW et al., eds. *Health impact, identification, and dosimetry of irradiated foods. Report of a WHO Working Group.* Neuherberg, Institut für Strahlenhygiene des Bundesgesundheitsamtes (ISH-125), pp. 190–206.

Heide L, Bögl W (1988d) Thermoluminescence and chemiluminescence measurements as routine methods for the identification of irradiated spices. In: Bögl KW et al., eds. *Health impact, identification, and dosimetry of irradiated foods. Report of a WHO Working Group.* Neuherberg, Institut für Strahlenhygiene des Bundesgesundheitsamtes (ISH-125), pp. 207–232.

Heide L, Bögl KW (1989) Nachweis der Bestrahlung an Erdbeeren durch Thermolumineszenzmessung. [Detection of the irradiation of strawberries by measurement of thermoluminescence.] *Bundesgesundheitsblatt,* **32**:388.

Heide L, Bögl KW (1990) Detection methods for irradiated food—luminescence and viscosity measurements. *International journal of radiation biology,* **57**: 201–219.

Heide L et al. (1986a) *Ein erster Ringversuch zur Identifizierung strahlenbehandelter Gewürze mit Hilfe von Lumineszenzmessungen.* [*A first round-robin study of the identification of irradiated spices by means of luminescence measurements.*] Neuherberg, Institut für Strahlenhygiene des Bundesgesundheitsamtes (ISH-101).

Heide L et al. (1986b) Die Identifizierung bestrahlter Lebensmittel mit Hilfe von Lumineszenzmessungen. [Identification of irradiated foodstuffs by means of luminescence measurements.] *Bundesgesundheitsblatt,* **29**:51–56.

Heide L et al. (1987a) *Viskositätsmessung—ein Verfahren zur Identifizierung strahlenbehandelter Gewürze?* [*Measurement of viscosity—a method of identifying irradiated spices?*] Neuherberg, Institut für Strahlenhygiene des Bundesgesundheitsamtes (ISH-120).

Heide L et al. (1987b) *Thermolumineszenz- und Chemilumineszenzmessungen als Routine-methoden zur Identifizierung strahlenbehandelter Gewürze. Untersuchungen zur Festlegung von Grenzwerten für Unterscheidung bestrahlter von unbesstrahlten Proben.* [*Measurement of thermoluminescence and chemiluminescence as a routine method of identification of irradiated spices. Studies to determine limiting values for distinguishing between irradiated and nonirradiated samples.*] Neuherberg, Institut für Strahlenhygiene des Bundesgesundheitsamtes (ISH-109).

Heide L et al. (1988) Are viscosity measurements a suitable method for the identification of irradiated spices? In: Bögl KW et al., eds. *Health impact, identification, and dosimetry of irradiated foods. Report of a WHO Working Group.* Neuherberg, Institut für Strahlenhygiene des Bundesgesundheitsamtes (ISH-125), pp. 176–189.

Heide L et al. (1989a) *Thermolumineszenz- und Chemilumineszenzmessungen zur Identifizierung strahlenbehandelter Gewürze: ein europäischer Ringversuch.* [*Measurement of thermoluminescence and chemiluminescence for the identification of irradiated spices: a European round-robin study.*] Neuherberg, Institut für Strahlenhygiene des Bundesgesundheitsamtes (ISH-130).

Heide L et al. (1989b) Identification of irradiated spices with luminescence measurements: a European comparison. *Radiation physics and chemistry*, 34:903–913.

Hoey B et al. (1991) Detection of irradiation-induced modifications in foodstuff DNA using ^{32}P post-labeling. In: Raffi JJ, Belliardo JJ, eds. *Potential new methods of detection of irradiated food.* Luxembourg, Commission of the European Communities (BCR Workshop, EUR-13331).

IUPAC (1990) Harmonized protocols for the adoption of standardized analytical methods and for the presentation of their performance characteristics. *Pure and applied chemistry*, 62:149.

Jabir AW et al. (1989) DNA modifications as a means of detecting the irradiation of wheat. *Radiation physics and chemistry*, 34:935–940.

Jeffries DA (1983) *Detection of irradiated foods.* Leatherhead, Food Research Association (Literature Survey, No. 14).

Jona R, Fronda A (1990) Rapid differentiation between gamma irradiated and non-irradiated potato tubers. *Radiation physics and chemistry*, 35:317–320.

Kampelmacher EH (1988) Identification of irradiated foods by microbial control. In: Bögl KW et al., eds. *Health impact, identification, and dosimetry of irradiated foods. Report of a WHO Working Group.* Neuherberg, Institut für Strahlenhygiene des Bundesgesundheitsamtes (ISH-125), pp. 342–346.

Karam LR, Simic MG (1988a) Ortho-tyrosine as a marker in post irradiation dosimetry (PID) of chicken. In: Bögl KW et al., eds. *Health impact, identification, and dosimetry of irradiated foods. Report of a WHO Working Group.* Neuherberg, Institut für Strahlenhygiene des Bundesgesundheitsamtes (ISH-125), pp. 297–304.

Karam LR, Simic MG (1988b) Detecting irradiated foods: use of hydroxyl radical biomarkers. *Analytical chemistry*, 60:1117A–1119A.

Kawamura Y et al. (1989a) A half-embryo test for identification of gamma-irradiated grapefruit. *Journal of food science*, 54:379–382.

Kawamura Y et al. (1989b) Improvement of the half-embryo test for the detection of gamma-irradiated grapefruit and its application to irradiated oranges and lemons. *Journal of food science*, 54:1501–1504.

Kent M (1991) Thermal properties (DSC) of irradiated food. In: Raffi JJ, Belliardo JJ, eds. *Potential new methods of detection of irradiated food.* Luxembourg, Commission of the European Communties (BCR Workshop, EUR-13331).

Ladomery LG (1991) Methods for detection of irradiated foods. *The referee (Journal of the Association of Official Analytical Chemists)*, **15**:1.

Lea JS et al. (1988) A method of testing for irradiation of poultry. *International journal of food science and technology*, **23**:625–632.

Leonardi M et al., eds. (1992) *Recent advances in the detection of irradiated foods.* Luxembourg, Commission of the European Communities (EUR-14315).

Mahesh K, Vij DR, eds. (1985) *Techniques of radiation dosimetry.* New Delhi, Wiley Eastern Limited.

McWeeny DJ et al. (1990) Evaluation of the limulus amoebocyte lysate test in conjunction with a gram negative bacterial plate count for detecting irradiated chicken. *Radiation physics and chemistry*, **36**:629–638.

Meier W (1991) Working field and research program. In: Raffi JJ, Belliardo JJ, eds. *Potential new methods of detection of irradiated foods.* Luxembourg, Commission of the European Communities (BCR Workshop, EUR-13331).

Meier W et al. (1988) Analysis of o-tyrosine as a method for the identification of irradiated chicken meat. *Beta-gamma*, **1**:34–36.

Meier W et al. (1989) Nachweis von bestrahltem Frischfleisch (Poulet) mittels o-tyrosin. [Detection of irradiated fresh meat (chicken) by means of o-tyrosine.] *Mitteilungen aus dem Gebiete des Lebensmittelshygienes*, **80**:22–29.

Meier W et al. (1990) Analysis of o-tyrosine as a method for the identification of irradiated chicken and the comparison with other methods (analysis of volatiles and ESR spectroscopy). *Radiation physics and chemistry*, **35**:332–336.

Merritt C Jr (1984) *Radiolysis compounds in bacon and chicken* (PB-84-187095; available from National Technical Information Service, Springfield, VA, USA).

Merritt C Jr et al. (1985) A quantitative comparison of the yields of radiolytic products in various meats and their relationship to precursors. *Journal of the American Oil Chemists Society,* **62**:708.

Merritt C Jr, Taub IA (1983) Commonality and predictability of radiolytic products in irradiated meats In: Elias PS, Cohen AJ, eds. *Recent advances in food irradiation.* Amsterdam, Elsevier Biomedical, pp. 27–57.

Mitchell GE (1987) Methods for the detection of irradiated food. In: *Food irradiation 1987. Proceedings of the Food Irradiation Session of the 56th Congress of* the *Australian and New Zealand Association for the Advancement of Science*, pp. 24–37.

Mohr E, Wichman G (1985) Viskositätserniedrigung als Indiz einer Cobaltbestrahlung von Gewürzen. [Reduction of viscosity as indicator of cobalt irradiation of spices.] *Gordian*, **85**:96.

Morehouse KM, Desrosiers MF (1993) Electron spin resonance investigations of gamma-irradiated shrimp shell. *Applied radiation and isotopes*, **44**:429–432.

Morehouse KM, Ku Y (1990) A gas chromatographic method for the identification of irradiated frog legs. *Radiation physics and chemistry*, **35**:337–341.

Morehouse KM, Ku Y (1992) Gas chromatographic and electron spin resonance investigations of gamma-irradiated shrimp. *Journal of agricultural and food chemistry*, **40**:1963–1971.

Morehouse KM et al. (1991) Gas chromatographic and electron spin resonance investigations of gamma-irradiated frog legs. *Radiation physics and chemistry*, **38**:61–68.

Moriarty TF et al. (1988) Thermoluminescence in irradiated foodstuffs. *Nature*, **332**:22.

Morishita N et al. (1988) Identification of irradiated pepper by ESR measurement. *Food irradiation, Japan*, **23**:28.

Nawar WW (1983a) Comparison of chemical consequences of heat and irradiation treatment of lipids. In: Elias PS, Cohen AJ, eds. *Recent advances in food irradiation*. Amsterdam, Elsevier Biomedical, pp. 115–127.

Nawar WW (1983b) Radiolysis of nonaqueous components of foods. In: Josephson ES, Peterson MS, eds. *Preservation of food by ionizing radiation*. Boca Raton, FL, CRC Press, Vol. 2, pp. 75–124.

Nawar WW (1986) Volatiles from food irradiation. *Food reviews international*, **21**:45–78.

Nawar WW (1988) Analysis of volatiles as a method for the identification of irradiated foods. In: Bögl KW et al., eds. *Health impact, identification, and dosimetry of irradiated foods. Report of a WHO Working Group*. Neuherberg, Institut für Strahlenhygiene des Bundesgesundheitsamtes, pp. 287–296 (ISH-125).

Nawar WW, Balboni JJ (1970) Detection of irradiation treatment in foods. *Journal of the Association of Official Analytical Chemists*, **53**:726–729.

Oestling O, von Hofsten B (1988) Health impact. In: Bögl KW et al., eds. *Health impact, identification, and dosimetry of irradiated foods. Report of a WHO Working Group*. Neuherberg, Institut für Strahlenhygiene des Bundesgesundheitsamtes (ISH-125), pp. 305–307.

Onderdelinden D, Strackee L (1974) ESR as a tool for the identification of irradiated foodstuffs. In: *The identification of irradiated foodstuffs*. Luxembourg, Commission of the European Communities, pp. 127–140.

Parsons B (1987) Prospective methods for testing the irradiation of foods. *Food science and technology today*, 1:148–150.

Pfeilsticker K, Lucas J (1987) Die fluorimetrische Bestimmung von Thyminglycol in Lebensmitteln (biologischem Material)—der Thyminglycolgehalt als Kriterium für eine Behandlung mit ionisierenden Strahlen. [The fluorimetric determination of thymine glycol in foodstuffs (biological material)—the thymine glycol content as criterion of treatment with ionizing radiation.] *Angewandte Chemie*, 99:341.

Qi Shengchu et al. (1990) Detection of irradiated liquor. *Radiation physics and chemistry*, 35:329–331.

Raffi JJ (1991) General introduction. In: Raffi JJ, Belliardo JJ, eds. *Potential new methods of detection of irradiated food*. Luxembourg, Commission of the European Communities (BCR Workshop, EUR-13331).

Raffi JJ Agnel JPL (1989) Electron spin resonance of irradiated fruits. *Radiation physics and chemistry*, 34:891–894.

Raffi JJ et al. (1987) Identification par résonance paramagnetique électronique de céréals irradiés. *Sciences des aliments*, 7:657–663.

Raffi JJ et al. (1988) Electron spin resonance identification of irradiated strawberries. *Journal of the Chemical Society, Faraday transactions I*, 84:3359.

Raffi JJ et al. (1989) ESR analysis of irradiated frog's legs and fishes. *International journal of applied radiation and isotopes*, 40:1215.

Raffi JJ et al. (1993) *Concerted action of the Community Bureau of Reference on methods of identification of irradiated foods. Final report*. Luxembourg, Commission of the European Communities.

Rhee JS (1969) *Apparent viscosity of shrimp homogenate as a quality index of shrimp irradiated at cryogenic temperatures*. Baton Rouge, Louisiana State University [Dissertation].

Rustichelli F (1991) Use of differential scanning calorimetry (DSC) for the identification of irradiated poultry meat. In: Raffi JJ, Belliardo JJ, eds. *Potential new methods of detection of irradiated food*. Luxembourg, Commission of the European Communities (BCR Workshop, EUR-13331).

Sanderson DCW (1990) In: Johnston DE, Stevenson MH, eds. *Food irradiation and the chemist*. Cambridge, Royal Society of Chemistry, pp. 25–56.

Sanderson DCW (1991) Photostimulated luminescence (PSL): a new approach to identifying irradiated foods. In: Raffi JJ, Belliardo JJ, eds. *Potential new methods of detection of irradiated food*. Luxembourg, Commission of the European Communities (BCR Workshop, EUR-13331).

Sanderson DCW et al. (1989a) Thermoluminescence of foods: origins and implications for detecting irradiation. *Radiation physics and chemistry*, **34**:915–924.

Sanderson DCW et al. (1989b) Detection of irradiated food. *Nature*, **340**:23.

Schellenberg KA, Shaeffer J (1986) Formation of methyl ester of 2-methyl glyceric acid from thymine glycol residues: a convenient new method for determining radiation damage to DNA. *Biochemistry*, **25**:1479.

Shieh JJ, Wierbicki E (1985) Interaction of radiation generated free radicals with collagen and metallo-proteins using cesium-137 gamma source. *Radiation physics and chemistry*, **25**:155–165.

Simic MG, de Graff E (1981) Radiation chemistry. Principles for commercial food applications. *Food development*, November, pp. 54–62, 66.

Simic MG et al. (1983) Radiation chemistry—extravaganza or an internal component of radiation processing of food. *Radiation physics and chemistry*, **22**:233–242.

Simic MG et al. (1985) Kinetics and mechanisms of hydroxyl radical-induced cross-links between phenylalanine peptides. *Radiation physics and chemistry*, **24**:465.

Sjöberg AM et al. (1990a) Detecting irradiation treatment of foods and spices. *Kemia-Kemi*, **17**:1033.

Sjöberg AM et al. (1990b) Nachweisverfahren für die Bestrahlung von Gewürzen. *Zeitschrift für Lebensmittel-Untersuchung und -Forschung*, **190**:99–103.

Sjöberg AM et al. (1993) Microbiological screening method for indication of irradiation of spices and herbs: a BCR collaborative study. *Journal of the Association of Official Analytical Chemists* **76**:674–681.

Solar S (1985) Reaction of hydroxyl radical with phenylalanine in neutral aqueous solution. *Radiation physics and chemistry*, **26**:103–109.

Spano M (1991) Use of flow cytometry for the possible identification of radio-induced changes in DNA of animal cells. In: Raffi JJ, Belliardo JJ, eds. *Potential new methods of detection of irradiated food*. Luxembourg, Commission of the European Communities (BCR Workshop, EUR-13331).

Sparenberg H (1974) Identificatie van bestraalde aardappelen. [Identification of irradiated potatoes.] In: *The identification of irradiated foodstuffs. Proceedings of an international conference*. Luxembourg, Commission of the European Communities, p. 325.

Stachowicz W et al. (1992) Application of electron paramagnetic resonance (EPR) spectroscopy for control of irradiated food. *Journal of the science of food and agriculture*, **58**:407–415.

Stevenson MH (1991) The use of 2-alkylcyclobutanones for the detection of irradiated food. In: Raffi JJ, Belliardo JJ, eds. *Potential new methods of detection of irradiated food*. Luxembourg, Commission of the European Communities. (BCR Workshop, EUR-13331).

Stevenson MH (1992) Progress in the identification of irradiated foods. *Trends in food science and technology*, **3**:257–262.

Stevenson MH, Gray R (1989) An investigation into the effect of sample preparation methods on the resulting ESR signal from irradiated chicken bone. *Journal of the science of food and agriculture*, **46**:262–267.

Suzuki T et al. (1988) Dosimetric application of near infrared spectroscopy to irradiated spices. *Food irradiation, Japan*, **23**:77.

Swallow AJ (1988) Some approaches based on radiation chemistry for identifying irradiated food. In: Bögl KW et al., eds. *Health impact, identification, and dosimetry of irradiated foods, Report of a WHO Working Group*. Neuherberg, Institut für Strahlenhygiene des Bundesgesundheitsamtes, pp. 128–138 (ISH-125).

Thayer DW (1988) Residual thiamin analysis for the identification of irradiated foods. In: Bögl KW et al., eds. *Health impact, identification, and dosimetry of irradiated foods. Report of a WHO Working Group*. Neuherberg, Institut für Strahlenhygiene des Bundesgesundheitsamtes (ISH-125), pp. 313–319.

Tuominen J (1991) Volatile decomposition products of lipids for detection of irradiated food. In: Raffi JJ, Belliardo JJ, eds. *Potential new methods of detection of irradiated food*. Luxembourg, Commission of the European Communities (BCR Workshop, EUR-13331).

Vajdi M, Merritt C Jr (1985) Identification of adduct radiolysis products from pork fat. *Journal of the American Oil Chemists Society*, **62**:1252.

van Spreekens KJA, Toepoel L (1978) Detection of irradiation in prepacked fresh fish and shrimps on the basis of the microbial flora. In: *Food preservation by irradiation. Proceedings of an international conference*. Vol. II. Vienna, International Atomic Energy Agency, pp. 157–170.

von Sonntag C (1987) *The chemical basis of radiation biology*. London, Taylor and Francis.

von Sonntag C (1988) Some considerations for developing analytical methods detecting the irradiation of food. In: Bögl KW et al., eds. *Health impact, identification, and dosimetry of irradiated foods. Report of a WHO Working Group*. Neuherberg, Institut für Strahlenhygiene des Bundesgesundheitsamtes, pp. 269–280 (ISH-125).

Wang D, von Sonntag C (1991) Radiation-induced oxidation of phenylalanine. In: Raffi JJ, Belliardo JJ, eds. *Potential new methods of detection of irradiated food.* Luxembourg, Commission of the European Communities (BCR Workshop, EUR-13331), p. 207.

Wichmann G et al. (1990) Optimierte Viskossitätsmessung zum Nachweis der Behandlung von Gewürzen mit Co^{60}-gamma-strahlen. [Optimized viscosity measurement for detection of treatment of spices with Co^{60} gamma radiation.] *Gordian,* **90**:8–13.

Yang GC et al. (1987) An ESR study of free radicals generated by gamma-irradiation of dried spices and spray-dried fruit powders. *Journal of food quality,* **10**: 287–294.

Zehnder HJ (1984) Zur Strahlenkonservierung von Zwiebeln. Versuche 1977–1983. [On the preservation of onions by irradiation. Studies 1977–1983.] *Alimenta,* **23**:114.

Zehnder HJ (1988) Nachweis bestrahlter Champignons (*Agaricus bisporus*)–theorie und praxis. *Mitteilungen aus dem Gebiete der Lebensmitteluntersuchung und Hygiene,* **79**:362–370.

6.
Toxicology

6.1 Introduction

Several hundred toxicological studies have been conducted on experimental animals over the past four decades. A variety of foods irradiated at different doses have been fed to rats, mice, dogs, monkeys, hamsters and pigs in order to assess all possible toxicological effects. The database is impressive by virtue of the sheer number of studies that have been conducted.

The question is whether this large database is adequate to demonstrate the safety of irradiated food for human consumption under specified conditions of use. An important aspect of this issue is the extent to which studies on one particular food type can be extrapolated to others. For instance, can the results of the studies on fish be extrapolated to beef or chicken, and to what extent do studies on strawberries bear any relationship to those on wheat? In other words, should there be one large database on all irradiated food or many small databases on different types of food? Similarly, are the radiolytic products formed by one type of radiation the same as those formed by other types, and to what extent do such products change qualitatively when higher doses are applied? The answers to these questions depend on an understanding of the nature and chemistry of irradiated food (see Chapters 4 and 5). Those aspects relevant to the adequacy of the toxicology database to demonstrate the safety of irradiated food are summarized below.

Food consists essentially of three macronutrients—protein, carbohydrate and fat. Meat, poultry and fish are high in protein and fat content and virtually devoid of carbohydrates. Vegetables and grains are high in carbohydrate content but tend to be relatively low in fat and protein. As explained in Chapter 4, the vast bulk of radiolytic products will be derived from the macronutrients. Consequently, the levels and patterns of radiolytic products in irradiated food will vary, depending on the macronutrient composition. From a toxicological point of view, foods of animal origin such as beef, pork, horse meat, chicken and even fish are quite similar in macronutrient composition and data on them can therefore be viewed as constituting a single database. Similarly, plant products such as vegetables and grains are similar in terms of macronutrient composition, and data on them can also be viewed as constituting a single database. As pointed out in Chapter 4, the quantity of radiolytic products formed increases linearly with the applied dose regardless of the dose rate or the source of radiation. In addition, it needs to be borne in mind that foods irradiated in the frozen state will have far fewer radiolytic products than those irradiated at room temperature. The levels of radiolytic products formed can also be reduced by irradiating food anaerobically or in the presence of antioxidants.

6.2 Toxicity studies

6.2.1 Studies in the FDA electronic database

Following the 1981 report of the Joint FAO/IAEA/WHO Expert Committee on the Wholesomeness of Irradiated Food, the FDA began a systematic review of the over 400 studies on toxicology available up to 1982. Of these, over 250 were "accepted" or "accepted with reservation", about 150 were "rejected" and more than 20 others were not categorized because they were review articles (Food and Drug Administration, 1986).

Studies were "rejected" on the following grounds:

- the radiation dose was not reported;
- the radiation dose was less than 0.1 kGy or more than 100 kGy;
- the number of animals used per group was not reported;
- in studies on rodents, the number of animals per group was less than five;
- the diet fed was determined to be nutritionally inadequate;
- the study was conducted without controls fed a nonirradiated diet;
- the irradiated food was not administered orally;
- the type of food irradiated was not reported;
- the studies were conducted at a laboratory that was considered by the FDA to be in violation of good laboratory practice.

Studies that were considered to have deficiencies that interfered with the interpretation of the data were "accepted with reservation" provided that none of the defects noted above were present. The position taken by the FDA was that such studies, while not able to stand alone, could provide important information for use in combination with others. It should be emphasized that the deficiencies were not the same in all the studies but varied. If, for example, 10 or more studies, each with different individual deficiencies, all indicated the absence of treatment-related toxicological effects, that would be compelling evidence that such effects were not occurring.

Studies were "accepted" if on initial examination they appeared to be reasonably complete. Such studies were given the designation "A", those accepted with reservation were designated "B", and those which were rejected because they failed to satisfy one or more of the criteria listed above were designated "R".

After further review, the FDA determined that many of the studies designated as "A" also contained minor deficiencies. For both "A" and "B" studies, the deficiencies can be divided into two major groups, as follows:

1. *Dietary problems*

    - Micronutrient (vitamin, mineral, etc.) or macronutrient (protein) deficiency.
    - Reduced or restricted food intake for any reason.
    - Unpalatable diets, e.g. as a result of increased peroxidation of oils.

2. *Inadequate experimental design*

    - Inadequate control diet.
    - Too few animals per group.
    - Use of animals of only one sex.
    - Combination of data in inappropriate ways, e.g. reporting only total number of tumours.
    - Inadequate presentation of data for evaluation, e.g. only in the form of a summary.
    - Addition of antioxidants such as butylated hydroxyanisole, butylated hydroxytoluene or ethoxyquin to the diet, either before or after irradiation.
    - Insufficient recovery time between breedings allowed for female animals in a reproductive study.
    - Animals not selected or assigned to groups at random.
    - Questionable culling practices in reproduction studies.
    - Inadequate histopathology.
    - Duration of study inadequate, e.g. for assessing carcinogenicity.
    - Inclusion of additional animals in the course of the study.

Despite the presence of minor or major deficiencies in many of the studies reviewed, the general absence of toxicological effects in such a large number of studies is impressive. The individual toxicological studies and tests reported, including subchronic studies in multiple species, chronic studies in multiple species, reproductive studies in multiple species and a series of mutagenicity tests, are discussed below. In general, these are of the type on which both the FDA and WHO rely in judging food safety (Food and Drug Administration, 1982; WHO, 1987). It should also be mentioned that the findings were similar in nature in all the studies, whether designated as A, B, or R. There is, for instance, no indication that R studies report effects not observed in A or B studies and attributed either to design problems or secondary nutritional effects, nor is there a greater percentage of claimed effects in R studies. Of over 40 reproduction studies, for example, 17 were placed in the R class and, of these, three reported effects. Although the effects reported were different in each of the studies, they were, however, similar to those reported in A and B studies, of which there were also three that claimed effects.

Subchronic studies

A total of 26 subchronic studies in the rat were designated as either A or B, as shown in Table 4. These covered a wide variety of foods, including onions, fish, pork, bread, beans, fruit, potatoes, shrimp, beef, bacon, and mushrooms. Radiation doses ranged from 0.1 kGy to 55.8 kGy. While a few effects were reported, the vast majority of the studies were negative, indicating a lack of any toxicological response to the consumption of irradiated food. An explanation of the few effects seen is given below.

In a study by Brin et al. (1961a), pork irradiated at a dose of 55.8 kGy and fed to rats for 84 days led to a decrease in serum alanine aminotransferase and a reduction in body weight. As indicated by the authors, these effects were probably due to the destruction of pyridoxine. The study was viewed by the FDA as a nutrition study and the findings as having no toxicological significance. Malhotra & Reber (1963a), reported the occurrence of haemorrhagic diathesis in rats fed beef irradiated at 55.8 kGy, a dose at which vitamin K is destroyed. Such losses are of little consequence for humans because beef is a relatively poor source of this vitamin. Since the diet fed to the rats was already deficient in vitamin K, its destruction by irradiation led to the haemorrhagic condition, which was not caused by toxic substances in the irradiated beef. Metwalli (1977) reported a significant decrease in serum aspartate aminotransferase activity in female rats whose whole diet was irradiated at 25 and 45 kGy. The FDA viewed this result as questionable because of the lack of a dose–response relationship. It was of only marginal statistical significance and might have been due to the enzyme activity in the controls being higher than typical.

Luckey et al. (1973) reported that mice fed an irradiated diet (54 kGy) appeared to grow more slowly and exhibited signs of anaemia. The FDA rejected this study for the following reasons:

1. The nonirradiated diet (control diet) was deficient in phosphorus, calcium, iron, copper, cobalt, manganese, riboflavin, thiamine, pyridoxine, pantothenate and folate. Irradiation at 54 kGy results in slight losses of riboflavin, pyridoxine and pantothenate, exacerbating the existing deficiencies.
2. The inadequacy of the control diet was demonstrated by the failure of the mice to gain weight as expected. At 42 days of age their weight was only 70% of that of mice on control laboratory chow diets.
3. The mice on an irradiated diet and raised in bioisolation grew more slowly than mice on a nonirradiated control diet, and more slowly than mice on an irradiated diet but reared in the open laboratory during the first generation. This situation, however, reversed itself in the second and third

6. TOXICOLOGY

Table 4. Subchronic toxicity studies in rats

Food	Duration (days)	Dose (kGy)	Effect	Class	Reference
Fish (mackerel)	90	2	None	B	Aravindakshan & Sundaram (1978)
Coffee, black beans	84	1	None	B	Bernardes (1980)
Pork	84	55.8	Body weight and serum alanine aminotransferase decreased	B	Brin et al. (1961a)
Pork, bread, beans, shrimps	84	55.8	None	B	Brin et al. (1961c)
Carrots	90	1	None	A	Coquet et al. (1980)
Chicken	90	6	None	A	de Knecht-van Echelen et al. (1971)
Fish (European plaice)	90	3.4	None	A	Inveresk Research International (1976)
Fish (cod, saithe)	84	3.4	None	A	Dent et al. (1977)
Mangoes	90	0.8	None	A	Raltech Scientific Services (1979)
Onions	90	0.25	None	B	Gabriel & Edmonds (1976b)
Fish	90	6	None	A	Hickman et al. (1969b)
Fish (cod)	90	6	None	B	Hickman (1975a)
Potatoes	90	2	None	B	Jaarma & Henricson (1964)
Beef	90	55.8	Haemorrhagic deaths	B	Malhotra & Reber (1963a)
Beef	98	55.8	Increased prothrombin time	B	Malhotra et al. (1965)
Chicken	90	47	None	B	McGown et al. (1979)
Whole diet	120	45	Decreased serum aspartate aminotransferase	B	Metwalli (1977)
Fish (mackerel)	90	1.5	None	B	Nadharni (1980)
Beef, pork	84	55.8	Increased liver enzyme levels	B	Read et al. (1959)
Mix: beef, fish, bacon	84	60	None	B	Read & Kraybill (1958)
Cocoa beans	126	0.5	None	B	Takyi & Ofori-Mensah (1981)
Wheat	105	2	None	B	Vakil (1975c)
Mushrooms	90	5	None	B	van Logten et al. (1971)
Shrimps	90	3	None	B	van Logten et al. (1972)
Whole diet	90	50	None	B	van Logten et al. (1978)
Strawberries	90	50	Decreased growth	B	Verschuuren et al. (1966)

Table 5. Subchronic studies in mice and dogs

Food	Duration (days)	Dose (kGy)	Effect	Species	Class	Reference
Onions	90	0.1	None	Mouse	B	Aravindakshan et al. (1977)
Fish (carp), shrimps	90	2.5	None	Mouse	B	Hossain (1979)
Onions	90	0.25	Anaemia	Dog	B	Gabriel & Edmonds (1976a)
Fruits: cherries	90	4	None	Dog	B	Gabriel & Edmonds (1977b)
Beef	188	55.8	None	Dog	B	Reber et al. (1960)
Wheat flour	168	0.74	None	Dog	B	Reber et al. (1959)
Meat: beef, mutton	130	0.07	None	Dog	B	Wasserman & Trum (1955)
Potatoes	90	2	None	Dog	B	Jaarma & Henricson (1964)

generations, when mice reared on an irradiated diet in bioisolation became heavier than controls.

4. The laboratory in which the study was conducted had serious problems with fertility. Mice reared on untreated lab chow produced only seven litters from 12 female matings. Mice on autoclaved chow had only five litters from 12 female matings and mice fed the special Apollo diet (non-irradiated) produced only two litters from 12 female matings.
5. The haematological findings of the study, in particular the low white blood cell count and low haemoglobin, indicate the inadequacy of the Apollo diet.
6. The inadequacy of the Apollo diet for mice and other irregularities in the protocol render the results of this study uninterpretable.

Five of the six studies in dogs listed in Table 5 demonstrated no adverse effects. The foods fed were fruit irradiated at 4 kGy, beef irradiated at 55.8 kGy, wheat flour at 0.74 kGy, beef and mutton irradiated at 0.07 kGy and potatoes irradiated at 2 kGy. Gabriel & Edmonds (1976a) reported a variety of effects in dogs fed a diet containing 10% irradiated onions (dry weight), but the FDA concluded that they were not related to treatment, and pointed out that the number of animals per sex per group was too small for adequate evaluation. It should also be noted that no adverse effects were observed in the dog studies where higher levels of radiation were used. No adverse effects were seen in the mouse studies listed in Table 5.

Table 6. Reproduction and teratology studies in rats

Food	Duration (days)	Dose (kGy)	Effect	Class	Reference
Pork	730	55.8	None	B	Bubl (1961)
Potatoes	730	0.4	None	B	Burns & Abrams (1961)
Mixed spices	10	15	None	B	Lorand Eötvös University of Sciences and Central Food Research Institute (1979)
Wheat	160	2	None	A	Hickman et al. (1964)
Fish	40	6	None	B	Hickman et al. (1969a)
Oranges	160	2.79	Decreased weight gain	B	Phillips et al. (1961b)
Chicken, green beans	120	59	None	B	Richardson (1960)
Fish	120	6	Testicular atrophy, estrous cycles prolonged	B	Shillinger & Osipova (1970)
Onions	120	1	None	B	van Petten et al. (1966)
Fish	V	2	None	B	Zaitsev (1980)

V = number of days varied.

Reproduction and teratology studies

A total of 11 reproductive studies carried out in rats were reviewed, as indicated in Table 6. The meat fed included pork irradiated at 55.8 kGy, chicken irradiated at 59 kGy, and fish irradiated at 6 kGy. The vegetables fed included onions irradiated at 1 kGy, potatoes irradiated at 0.4 kGy, and green beans irradiated at 56 kGy. The grains included wheat irradiated at 2 kGy. One fruit, oranges, was irradiated at 2.79 kGy. Most of these studies were negative. In the study of irradiated fish by Shillinger & Osipova (1970), testicular atrophy and prolonged estrous cycles were noted, together with a 42% reduction in blood cholinesterase activity, indicating protein deficiency; the latter may be due either to reduced intake or to decreased wholesomeness of the fish. The diet appeared inadequate and no vitamin or mineral supplements were provided. The indices of reproductive function were questionable, no data being presented on the offspring, births, number of stillbirths, survival rates or organ weights despite reference being made to these parameters in the text. It was concluded that the data from this study were of doubtful value. The decreased weight gain seen by Phillips et al.

Table 7. Reproduction and teratology studies in mice

Food	Duration (days)	Dose (kGy)	Effect	Class	Reference
Maize, nuts, prunes	240	2	None	B	Baev (1980)
Whole diet	200	25	Decrease in number of litters	B	Porter & Festing (1970)
Chicken	20	59	None	B	Raltech Scientific Services (1983)
Chicken	V	45	None	B	Ronning (1980)
Chicken	18	45	None	B	Thomson et al. (1977)
Fish (cod, ocean perch)	120	1.75	None	A	Huntingdon Research Centre (1978)

V = number of days varied.

Table 8. Reproduction and teratology studies in dogs, hamsters and rabbits

Food	Duration (days)	Dose (kGy)	Effect	Species	Class	Reference
Beef	V	55.8	None	Dog	B	Clarkson & Pick (1964)
Chicken	5	45	None	Hamster	A	Dahlgren et al. (1977)
Chicken	14	45	None	Rabbit	A	Dahlgren et al. (1980)
Beef	900	56	None	Dog	A	Loosli et al. (1964)
Potatoes	V	0.15	None	Dog	B	McCay & Rumsey (1961)

V = number of days varied.

(1961b) was not considered to be related to treatment, and may have been due to dietary inadequacy.

Five reproductive studies were conducted in mice fed irradiated chicken (45 kGy), fish (1.75 kGy), maize, nuts and prunes (2 kGy), and whole diet (25 kGy) (Table 7). The only adverse effect reported was a smaller number of litters in the whole diet study (Porter & Festing, 1970), but this was not statistically significant.

Two reproductive studies were conducted in dogs fed irradiated beef at 56 kGy, no effect being observed in either study (Table 8). A third study in dogs fed potatoes irradiated at a much lower dose was also negative. One study was conducted in hamsters fed chicken irradiated at 45 kGy and another in rabbits fed chicken irradiated at the same dose. No adverse effects were detected in either study.

In summary, the reproduction and teratology studies conducted were overwhelmingly negative. The only adverse effects reported were either not statistically significant or could be explained by other factors.

Chronic toxicity studies

A total of 32 chronic studies carried out on rats were reviewed (Table 9). The duration of six of them was less than 600 days, but that of the remaining 26 studies was long enough for a proper assessment of carcinogenicity to be made. No treatment-related increase in tumours was seen in any of the studies, many of which involved feeding food irradiated at extremely high doses. Three studies involved feeding pork, either alone or with other foods, at doses of between 27.9 kGy and 74 kGy. No adverse effects were observed. In three studies, beef irradiated at doses ranging from 27.9 kGy to 55.8 kGy was fed, and again, no adverse effects were noted. Irradiated chicken was used in two studies. In that by Phillips et al. (1961), weanling rats were found to have reduced levels of alkaline phosphatase in their duodenal tissue, but there were only five animals of each sex in each dosage group, which was too few for an adequate evaluation of the data. No significant toxicological findings were observed in the rats fed the irradiated chicken stew and cabbage over their lifetime or in the two subsequent generations.

Chronic studies were also carried out using either a mixture of irradiated foods or whole diet. In one study in which bacon, ham, fish and other foods were mixed and irradiated at 55.8 kGy, Read et al. (1961) reported a decreased weight gain in the third generation, and significantly lower weanling weights in the second breeding of parents in both the second and third generations. However, the observed effect was small and it was not possible to determine whether the reduction in weight occurred during lactation or *in utero* because neither birth weights nor maternal weights were given. However, body weights became equal after weaning so that the effect observed was probably lactational. The decreased reproductive performance in controls and experimental groups in the second breeding is probably attributable to the females not having been given enough recovery time between breedings.

A total of 18 chronic studies were carried out on mice (Table 10). Mixtures of pork and chicken, pork and beef, beef, pork and fish, and tuna fish and beef were irradiated at doses from 27.9 kGy to 93 kGy without adverse effect. Bacon and bacon fat were irradiated at 55.8 kGy, chicken at 7 kGy in two studies, starch at 6 kGy and wheat flour at 2 kGy, no adverse effects being observed following lifetime feeding. Adverse effects were reported

Table 9. Chronic studies in rats

Food	Duration (days)	Dose (kGy)	Effect	Class	Reference
Bananas	730	0.4	None	B	Anon (1976a)
Fish (mackerel)	730	2	None	B	Anukaranhanonta et al. (1980)
Whole diet	728	25	None	B	Aravindakshan et al. (1978)
Beef	730	55.8	None	B	Bone (1963)
Pork, peach, flour, carrots	730	55.6	None	B	Bone (1963)
Potatoes	730	0.4	None	B	Brownell et al. (1959)
Chicken	730	6	None	A	de Knecht-van Echelen et al. (1972)
Mangoes	730	0.8	None	A	Raltech Scientific Services (1981)
Wheat	750	2	None	B	Hickman et al. (1964)
Fish	730	6	None	B	Hickman et al. (1969c)
Horse meat	630	6.5	None	B	Hickman (1975b)
Wheat	730	2	None	B	Ikeda et al. (1969)
Potatoes	730	0.6	None	B	Ikeda (1971)
Potatoes	455	2	None	B	Jaarma et al. (1966)
Strawberries	730	3	None	A	Nees (1970)
Potatoes	728	0.15	None	B	Huntingdon Research Centre (1975)
Corn, tuna fish	728	55.8	None	B	Paynter (1959)
Chicken stew/cabbage	730	56	Reduced levels of alkaline phosphatase in duodenal tissue	B	Phillips et al. (1961)

6. TOXICOLOGY

Food			Effect		Reference
Milk powder, beef stew	730	55.8	None	A	Radomski et al. (1965b)
Mix: bacon, ham, fish	721	55.8	Decreased weight gain in third generation	B	Read et al. (1961)
Milk powder	400	45	None	A	Renner & Reichelt (1973)
Potatoes	800	0.3	None	B	Shillinger & Kamaldinova (1973)
Mix: beef, pork, fish	365	27.9	None	B	Teply & Kline (1959)
Mix: pork, brain, beef	365	93	None	B	Teply & Kline (1959)
Oils: corn, cotton seed	365	55.8	None	B	Teply & Kline (1959)
Mix: bacon, beef, fish	960	58	None	A	Teply & Kline (1959)
Starch	742	6	None	B	Truhaut & Saint-Lèbe (1978)
Wheat flour	999	2	None	B	Vakil (1975c)
Shrimps	999	2.5	None	B	Vakil (1975b)
Pork	900	74	None	B	van Logten et al. (1983)
Mushrooms, powdered	365	5	None	B	Vlielander & Chappel (1968a)
Fish	880	2	None	B	Zaitsev et al. (1977)

Table 10. Chronic studies in mice

Food	Duration (days)	Dose (kGy)	Effect	Class	Reference
Whole diet	730	60	Decrease in growth and fertility	B	Biagini et al. (1967)
Wheat flour	800	50	Tumour, reduced viability	B	Bugyaki (1973)
Fish	560	1.75	None	A	Chaubey et al. (1978)
Chicken	730	59	None	B	Raltech Scientific Services (1983)
Bacon	750	55.8	None	B	Dixon et al. (1961)
Fish (cod, perch)	560	1.75	None	B	Huntingdon Research Centre (1979)
Potatoes	730	0.6	None	B	Ikeda (1971)
Bacon fat	500	55.8	None	B	McKee et al. (1959)
Mix: pork, chicken	800	55.8	Auricular dilatation	B	Monsen (1960)
Chicken	560	7	None	B	Proctor (1974)
Chicken	580	7	None	B	Proctor (1971)
Mix: tuna fish, beef	730	55.8	None	B	Radomski et al. (1965a)
Mix: beef, pork, fish	365	27.9	None	B	Teply & Kline (1959)
Mix: pork brain, beef	365	93	None	B	Teply & Kline (1959)
Oils: corn, cotton seed	365	55.8	None	B	Teply & Kline (1959)
Mix: pork, chicken	600	55.8	None	A	Thompson et al. (1963)
Starch	742	6	None	B	Truhaut & Saint-Lèbe (1978)
Wheat flour	999	2	None	B	Vakil (1975a)

only in four of the studies, namely those in which mice were fed whole diet irradiated at 60 kGy, wheat flour at 50 kGy, chicken at 59 kGy, and a mixture of pork and chicken at 55.8 kGy. The effects noted (Table 10) differed from study to study, so that each reported adverse effect was observed only once in the 18 mouse studies. Biagini et al. (1967) reported decreased growth and fertility in mice fed whole diets irradiated at 60 kGy, but the reduction in growth was less than 10% and the fertility problems appeared to be related to nutrition. Furthermore, the investigators failed to rotate the males to nonpregnant females, and there were palatability problems with the diet. Monsen (1960) suspected that a diet consisting of pork, chicken and other food irradiated at a dose of 55.8 kGy led to the development of auricular dilatation in the hearts of mice. However, a much larger study involving nearly 5000 mice of the same strain was conducted by Thompson et al. (1963) in Monsen's laboratory. Despite extensive and detailed histopathology of more than 800 000 heart tissue sections, no lesions of the type described were found, demonstrating that irradiation was not responsible for the heart lesions originally reported. The overall results of 18 chronic studies in mice show that a variety of irradiated food, including whole diet irradiated at high levels, have no adverse effects on the animals following lifetime feeding.

Table 11 lists 11 chronic studies conducted in dogs. Unlike those conducted in rats and mice, the duration of these studies was inadequate to enable tumorigenicity or carcinogenicity to be properly assessed. Three studies involved feeding chicken irradiated at doses ranging from 6 kGy to 59 kGy, two involved feeding beef irradiated at 55.8 kGy, and one involved feeding bacon and cabbage irradiated at 55.8 kGy. Other studies involved soft-shell clams irradiated at 8 kGy, onions at doses of 1 kGy or less, bananas at 4 kGy, strawberries at 3 kGy, and wheat flour at 0.74 kGy. Reber et al. (1961) reported thyroiditis when dogs were fed wheat flour irradiated at 0.74 kGy. However, only two dogs of each sex were included in each dosage group and the findings lack statistical significance. There were also difficulties in whelping, one litter in the control group and one in the low-dose group being lost. Furthermore, a large number of pups in both groups died before weaning, suggesting that there may have been a problem during lactation. The effect was not related to irradiation. As thyroiditis is relatively common in beagles, it is impossible to say that this effect was treatment-related. Overall, the 11 studies in dogs were generally negative and there

Table 11. Chronic studies in dogs

Food	Duration (days)	Dose (kGy)	Effect	Class	Reference
Bananas	730	4	None	B	Anon (1976b)
Chicken	999	59	None	B	Raltech Scientific Services (1982)
Chicken, beef, jam	730	55.8	None	B	Blood et al. (1966)
Clams, soft-shelled	728	8	Decrease in blood urea nitrogen	B	Fegley & Edmonds (1976)
Bacon, cabbage	730	55.8	None	B	Hale et al. (1960)
Onions	540	0.2	None	B	Hilliard et al. (1966)
Onions	540	1	None	B	Hilliard (1974)
Strawberries	730	3	None	B	Nees & Sharma (1970)
Wheat flour	730	0.74	Thyroiditis	B	Reber et al. (1961)
Beef	728	55.8	None	B	Reber et al. (1962)
Chicken	365	6	None	A	Til et al. (1971)

Table 12. Chronic studies in monkeys and pigs

Food	Duration (days)	Dose (kGy)	Effect	Species	Class	Reference
Potatoes	300	0.15	None	Pig	B	Jaarma & Bengtsson (1966)
Rice	730	1	None	Monkey	B	Tobe et al. (1980)

were no effects that appeared consistently or that showed any pattern or trend.

As indicated in Table 12, one study was conducted in pigs fed for 300 days with potatoes irradiated at 0.15 kGy and another in monkeys fed for 730 days with rice irradiated at 1 kGy. In neither study were any adverse effects observed.

In summary, over 30 chronic studies in rats, 18 in mice and 11 in dogs were conducted. In the majority of cases, food irradiated at high doses was fed for a lifetime or at least a year. No effects were seen showing any consistent pattern or trend, and the studies were overwhelmingly negative, indicating that the consumption of irradiated food, either over the lifetime of the animals or a significant fraction of it, had no toxicological effect.

Mutagenesis

Dominant lethal mutations

More than 20 of the studies listed in Table 13 were conducted to assess the potential of irradiated foods to induce dominant lethal mutations in rats and mice. The only A and B studies (see p. 82) that showed an increase in dominant lethal mutations were those conducted by Vijayalaxmi (1976) and Vijayalaxmi & Rao (1976). However, it seems most unlikely that the reported effect was due to feeding wheat irradiated at 0.75 kGy, since other studies using much higher doses were negative.

Polyploidy

A study of malnourished Indian children (Bhaskaram & Sadasivan, 1975) who consumed wheat irradiated at 0.75 kGy for 4–6 weeks has been the focus of enormous controversy. Five children were placed in each of three different groups; the first was fed freshly irradiated wheat, the second stored irradiated wheat, and the third nonirradiated wheat. Approximately 100 peripheral blood cells were counted for each child or 500 cells per group. The percentages of cells showing polyploidy in children fed freshly irradiated wheat for 4 or 6 weeks were 0.8 and 1.8% of cells, respectively. No polyploidy was observed after the first 2 weeks of feeding. The effect was much lower in children fed stored irradiated wheat; no polyploid cells were observed either in children fed nonirradiated wheat or in any of the children before they were placed on the test diets. The authors also reported that polyploidy declined to background levels by 16–24 weeks after cessation of feeding. The statistical power of the study was limited by the small number of cells scored, so that very few polyploid cells were actually observed.

The results were expressed in terms of the mean numbers of polyploid cells in each group, but the limited data presented indicated wide variability among the children; this may represent, in part at least, a small-numbers effect. For the group showing the highest frequency of polyploid cells (1.8%), only nine polyploid cells were seen in four of the five children (the fifth child showed no polyploidy). Typically, a normal individual will exhibit between 0.1% and 1% of polyploid cells among peripheral blood cells (Bradsky & Vryvaeva, 1977). Consequently, the number of polyploid cells found in each group examined does not appear unusually high. The observation that the frequency of polyploidy among children fed freshly irradiated food declined to background levels 16–24 weeks after cessation of feeding is in conflict with the fact that thymic lymphocytes persist in the circulation for many years, and suggests that the earlier observation was a chance phenomenon. The finding of no polyploid cells in the control group is also surprising, in view of reports of a high incidence of chromosomal aberrations in lymphocytes in malnourished children (Armendares et al., 1971).

The Indian Ministry of Health, in an effort to settle the controversy, established an expert committee in 1987 which reviewed in detail all the studies carried out at the Indian National Institute of Nutrition (NIN) and the Bhabha Atomic Research Centre (BARC) on the effects of irradiated wheat on various genetic and cytogenetic phenomena. The committee concluded that neither the design of the study nor the results were such as to demonstrate a treatment-related induction of polyploidy. In view of the weight of evidence of all the studies performed to date, it seems unlikely that the findings were the result of the consumption of irradiated wheat, and more probable that the slight differences observed occurred by chance. It should, in any case, be borne in mind that no significance can be attributed to polyploidy in terms of any specific disease.

A number of cytogenetic studies have been carried out in rodents fed wheat irradiated at 0.75 kGy. Vijayalaxmi & Sadasivan (1975) studied bone marrow cells in rats fed wheat within 20 days after irradiation. The animals were maintained on the diet for 12 weeks before their bone marrow underwent cytogenetic analysis. For 8 weeks before the experiment, half the animals were maintained on a low-protein diet (5%) and the remainder on a normal-protein diet (18%). Controls and groups fed irradiated wheat were subsequently maintained on the same low- or high-protein diets.

Table 13. Mutagenesis studies

Species	Food	Duration (days)	Dose (kGy)	Effect	Class	Reference
Mouse	Onions	5	0.1	None	B	Münzner & Renner (1981)
Rat	Onions, dehydrated	>	0.3	None	B	Anon (1980)
Rat	Fish (mackerel)	70	2.0	None	A	Anukaranhanonta et al. (1981)
Mouse	Onions	56	0.1	None	A	Aravindakshan et al. (1980)
Mouse	Maize, nuts, prunes	56	2.0	None	A	Baev et al. (1981)
Mouse	Black beans	56	0.5	None	A	Bernardes (1980)
Mouse	Black beans	56	20.0	None	A	Bernardes et al. (1981)
Human	Wheat	42	0.75	Increase in polyploid cells	B	Bhaskaram & Sadasivan (1975)
Vicia fab	Sugar solutions	>	20.0	Chromosome changes	A	Bradley et al. (1968)
Mouse	Cereals, onions, potatoes	7	3.0	None	B	Bronnikova & Okuneva (1973)
Mouse	Wheat	120	50.0	Chromosomal abnormalities in germ cells	A	Bugyaki et al. (1964)
Mouse	Fish (mackerel)	112	15.0	None	A	Chaubey et al. (1978)
Mouse	Whole diet	56	25.0	None	A	Chauhan et al. (1975b)
Rat	Whole diet	120	25.0	None	A	Chauhan et al. (1975a)
Rat	Wheat	84	0.75	None	A	Chauhan et al. (1977)
Barley, onion	Fruit juice	3	2.0	Chromosome breaks	A	Chopra et al. (1963)
Drosophila	Culture medium	>	10.0	None	A	Chopra (1965)
Rat	Mangoes	112	0.8	None	A	Derse (1978)
Rat	Mangoes	>	0.08	None	A	Derse (1979)
Rat	Mangoes	>	0.08	None	A	Derse (1979)
Rat	Whole diet	90	50.0	None	A	Eriksen & Emborg (1972)
Rat	Wheat, whole diet	56	0.75	None	A	George et al. (1976)
E. coli	Onions	>	0.30	None	A	Hattori et al. (1979)
Hamster	Chicken, fish, dates	6	7.0	None	A	Hofer et al. (1979)
Mouse	Fish (carp), shrimps	60	2.5	None	B	Hossain (1979)

Organism	Substrate	Dose	Effect	Reference	
Mouse	Fish (carp), shrimps	60	2.5	None	Hossain et al. (1981)	B
Human	Culture medium	V	5.0	Positive, cytogenetic	Kesavan & Swaminathan (1966)	B
Drosophila	DNA powder	5		None	Khan & Alderson (1965)	A
Mouse	Whole diet	30	25.0	None	Leonard et al. (1977)	B
Mouse	Potatoes	7	0.12	None	Levinsky et al. (1973)	A
Mouse	Potatoes	7	0.12	None	Levinsky & Wilson (1975)	A
Insects	Coffee, black beans	14	2.0	None	Loaharanu (1978)	B
Drosophila	Chicken	5	55.8	None	Lusskin (1979)	B
Drosophila	Onion	V	9.0	None	Mittler (1980)	A
Mouse	Whole diet	35	50.0	None	Moutschen-Dahmen et al. (1970)	A
Mouse	Potatoes	7	0.1	Positive mutations	Osipova (1974)	B
Mouse	Potatoes	7	0.1	Positive, cytogenetic	Osipova et al. (1975)	A
Rat	Potatoes	120	0.12	None	Palmer et al. (1973)	B
Mouse	Wheat	180	0.5	None	Reddi et al. (1972)	A
Mouse	Wheat flour	360	2.0	None	Reddi et al. (1977)	A
Rat/mouse	Milk powder	200	45.0	None	Renner et al. (1973)	A
Hamster	Whole diet	42	45.0	Polyploidy	Renner (1977)	A
Drosophila	Whole medium	12	5.0	None	Rinehart & Ratty (1965)	B
Drosophila	Whole medium	12	30.0	Sex-linked recessive lethal (SLRL) mutations	Rinehart & Ratty (1965)	B
Drosophila	Sucrose solution	V	30.0	None	Rinehart & Ratty (1967)	A
Vicia fab[a]	Strawberries	V	4.0	None	Ross et al. (1970)	A
Drosophila	Dates	5		None	Schlatter et al. (1980)	A
Mouse/rat	Strawberries	5	15.0	None	Schubert et al. (1973)	A
Human	Sucrose solution (2%)	3	20.0	Chromosome breaks	Shaw & Hayes (1966)	B
Barley embryos	Potato pulp	1	0.8	Positive micronuclei	Swaminathan et al. (1962)	A
Drosophila	Culture medium	5	1.5	SLRL mutations	Swaminathan et al. (1963)	B
Rat	Wheat	84	0.75	None	Tesh & Davidson (1976)	B
Rat	Wheat	84	0.75	Polyploidy	Vijayalaxmi (1975)	A
Mouse	Wheat	84	0.75	Polyploidy, dominant lethal mutations	Vijayalaxmi (1976)	B

Table 13 (continued)

Species	Food	Duration (days)	Dose (kGy)	Effect	Class	Reference
Monkey	Wheat	300	0.75	Polyploidy	B	Vijayalaxmi (1978)
Rat	Wheat	84	0.75	Dominant lethal mutations	B	Vijayalaxmi & Rao (1976)
Rat	Wheat	84	0.75	Polyploidy, chromosome breaks	B	Vijayalaxmi & Sadasivan (1975)
Hamster	Thymine	V	10.0	Sister chromatid exchange, chromosome breaks	B	Wills (1981)
Rat	Onions	7	0.1	None	A	Zaitsev (1980)
Rat/mouse	Potatoes	V	0.2	None	B	Zajcev et al. (1975)

V = number of days varied.

Chromosomal breaks and deletions were reported to be increased in animals fed the low-protein diet, but irradiation was not responsible for these structural chromosomal abnormalities. However, the authors reported a significant increase in the fraction of cells showing polyploidy in animals fed irradiated wheat, the protein content of the diet having no influence on this effect. A total of 3000 cells (500 cells per rat) were scored for polyploidy in each group of animals. If the irradiated wheat was stored for 3 months prior to feeding, no effect was observed. The frequency of polyploidy in control animals was extremely low in this study (0–0.05%). Although the levels rose to 0.4–0.7% in animals fed the irradiated diet, the numbers of polyploid cells scored were small and the results were statistically within the range observed by others in normal rat bone-marrow cells. In a similar study by Vijayalaxmi (1975), wheat irradiated at 0.75 kGy was fed to rats within 20 days of irradiation. No increase in the incidence of chromosome damage was seen, but an increased incidence of polyploidy was reported.

George et al. (1976) examined the frequency of polyploidy in bone marrow cells from Wistar rats fed wheat irradiated at 0.75 kGy. Rats were fed the wheat either 24 hours or 2 weeks after irradiation and maintained on the diet for 1 or 6 weeks before analysis of bone marrow cells. A number of experimental groups fed various proportions of wheat in the diet were examined. The mean frequency of polyploid cells varied between 0.2% and 0.3% in the five experimental and five control groups. There were no differences in the frequency of polyploid cells in rats fed nonirradiated as compared with irradiated wheat diets, even when the treated wheat was fed within 24 hours of irradiation. The study appears to have been well controlled, involving several variables which might influence the biological effect of irradiated food. It has considerably greater statistical power, as 3000 cells were scored per animal (as compared with 500 cells in the Vijayalaxmi & Sadasivan study) in a larger number of rats; about 40 polyploid cells were scored in each of the 12 experimental groups.

In a study by Tesh & Palmer (1980), aimed at resolving the question of polyploidy, 15 rats of each sex were fed either 70% wheat irradiated at 0.75 kGy (stored for 2 weeks before use) or nonirradiated wheat for a period of 12 weeks. No difference in the incidence of polyploidy was observed between the test and control groups. The micronucleus test was also performed on 10 of these same animals of each sex from each group, together with a dominant lethal study using four test groups and a control group of 15 male rats. No effects resulting from the ingestion of irradiated wheat were observed in any of these studies.

In a study on mice, Vijayalaxmi (1976) performed chromosome analyses of bone marrow cells on groups of two mice each fed 70% wheat, either non-irradiated or irradiated at 0.75 kGy, 2 weeks after irradiation or after storage for 3 months. The two mice fed freshly irradiated wheat were reported to have shown an increased incidence of polyploid cells. No effect was noted in the two mice fed irradiated wheat after storage.

Other mouse studies employing irradiated wheat failed to demonstrate an effect on the incidence of polyploidy in bone marrow cells. An investigation by Bronnikova & Okunera (1973) using irradiated wheat and other cereals found no difference between test and control groups with regard to chromosomal damage and polyploidy.

The Indian committee of experts, in its review of the data from studies carried out by NIN, including a review of the slides previously scored by NIN investigators and of rescored slides from both control and treated animals, did not find any evidence of an increased incidence of polyploid cells in the bone marrow of animals fed freshly irradiated wheat. The committee concluded that the apparent positive results were the result of inadequate sampling techniques. When NIN investigators were requested to rescore their own slides, the values obtained were very different from those reported earlier on the same slides. The re-analysis by the committee indicated that the frequency of polyploidy in control animals had been underestimated, whereas that in animals fed irradiated wheat had been overestimated. Furthermore, the error variance was large owing to bias in the selection of the portion of the slide to be sampled (central portion) as well as the inadequate size of the sample itself. BARC resolved these difficulties by sampling the cells over the entire slide, and scoring a larger number of metaphases. The committee concluded that the NIN and BARC studies were not inconsistent and that the data presented by NIN in support of an effect of irradiated wheat could not be confirmed.

Renner (1977) examined bone marrow cells from Chinese hamsters fed a diet sterilized by doses of 10–100 kGy. Animals were studied after periods of 24 hours or 6 weeks on the diet. No differences were observed in structural chromosomal aberrations but a 4–5-fold increase in the fraction of cells with polyploidy was found within 24 hours of feeding a diet irradiated with 45 kGy. When feeding was discontinued, the frequency of polyploid cells declined to control levels within 6 weeks. Furthermore, if the irradiated diet was stored initially for 6 weeks before feeding, no increase in polyploid cells was observed. Very high radiation doses were employed in this study. The effect was not dose-dependent over the range 30–100 kGy. The overall levels of polyploidy were extremely low, ranging from 0.06% in controls to 0.3% in animals fed irradiated diets. The effect was independent of whether the animals were fed the irradiated diet for 1 day or 6 weeks. Frohberg & Schulze Schencking (1975) have reported control levels of polyploidy in Chinese hamsters to be 0.31%. The suggestion by Renner (1977) that the increase in polyploidy could be due to hydrogen peroxide seems unlikely since, when fed in the diet, it would be subject to rapid breakdown by catalase well before reaching the bone marrow.

Vijayalaxmi (1978) also conducted cytogenetic studies on peripheral lymphocytes of monkeys fed 70% nonirradiated wheat, 70% freshly irradiated wheat (0.75 kGy) or 70% irradiated wheat (0.75 kGy) stored for more than 3 months. No differences were observed between groups in the incidence of chromosomal damage but an increase in polyploidy was reported in the group fed freshly irradiated wheat. This reported increase, like those reported by the same investigator for rats and mice, suffered from statistical inadequacy.

In conclusion, the group of studies discussed fails to provide convincing evidence that feeding wheat irradiated at 0.75 kGy produces karyotypic abnormalities in bone marrow cells or lymphocytes in a variety of mammalian species, or that irradiation of wheat at the same dose can induce polyploidy in malnourished children. The studies purporting to show an increase in polyploidy are all technically flawed; more careful analyses have indicated that their results are not significantly different from those of more comprehensive investigations that show no effect of irradiated wheat on polyploidy. The effects reported in the study in which higher radiation doses were used are also questionable. However, even in this study, no effect was observed at doses below 10 kGy or when food irradiated at higher doses was stored for 6 weeks.

Other mutagenicity studies

When pure solutions of glucose are irradiated, mutagenic compounds can be produced, and detected *in vitro* using appropriate strains in the Ames *Salmonella* test (Wilmer et al., 1981). Shaw & Hayes (1966) have demonstrated the induction of chromosomal breaks in human lymphocytes exposed to solutions of irradiated sucrose. Rinehart & Ratty (1965) have also shown the ability of irradiated glucose to induce mutations in *Drosophila melanogaster*. Such mutagenic effects, however, do not occur when food, which is a complex mixture, is irradiated, as shown in studies with *Salmonella typhimurium* in which irradiated fresh vegetables (van Kooij et al., 1978), onions (Hattori et al., 1979), fish (Joner et al., 1978), spices (Farkas et al., 1981) and chicken (Thayer et al., 1987) were used. In none of these studies were positive effects observed. Similarly, in studies with *Drosophila*, no increased mutagenicity was found for irradiated beef or ham (Mittler, 1979), dates (Renner et al., 1982) and onion powder (Mittler & Eiss, 1982).

As described in Chapter 5, chemical analytical studies have shown that mutagenic substances produced in simple sugar solutions do not occur in measurable amounts when the sugars are irradiated as constituents of fruits or fruit juices (den Drijver et al., 1986). It should also be noted that glucose irradiated either in solution (Aiyar & Rao, 1977; Schubert et al., 1967; Münzner & Renner, 1975) or in the dry state (Varma et al., 1986) did not exhibit any mutagenic effect when tested in mice or rats, nor did irradiated complex food induce chromosomal aberrations in bone marrow, micronuclei, or sister chromatid exchange in bone marrow and spermatogonia (Renner et al., 1982). As can be seen from Table 13, the great majority of studies indicate that the consumption of irradiated food does not result in mutations, dominant lethal effects or cytogenetic abnormalities.

6.2.2 Raltech studies

The studies described below, conducted at the Raltech Laboratory, are generally acknowledged as among the best and most statistically powerful of all the studies on food irradiation. Initially supported by the United States Army, then later by the US Department of Agriculture, these studies using irradiated chicken meat have now been completed and the reports are available from the National Technical Information Service in the USA. The studies required nearly a quarter of a million birds, or 134 tonnes of chicken meat. One of the studies, a mouse feeding study, was a combined carcinogenicity, chronic toxicity and multigeneration reproductive study.

Overall, the Raltech studies are among the most comprehensive ever conducted. In addition to the chronic feeding study in mice, they included a chronic feeding study in dogs, teratology studies in four species, a dominant lethal study in mice, a sex-linked recessive test in *Drosophila melanogaster* and an Ames mutagenicity test. In each animal feeding study, five groups of animals were used, fed as follows: (1) electron-irradiated chicken meat; (2) gamma-irradiated chicken meat; (3) heat-sterilized chicken meat; (4) enzyme-inactivated (blanched) chicken meat; (5) rodent or dog chow diet (control group). The mean radiation dose applied to the chicken meat fed to groups 1 and 2 was 58 kGy. Irradiation was carried out at $-25\,°C$ in the absence of air.

The teratology studies showed that feeding irradiated chicken meat to hamsters, rabbits, rats and mice did not result in teratogenic effects in offspring. The first three of these studies were considered by the FDA to be of high quality. The mouse teratology study, although negative, was considered by the FDA to be of limited value because of procedural flaws in recording the data (H. Irausquin, 1988, unpublished data).

The dominant lethal test in mice did not show any treatment-related effects in animals fed irradiated chicken. However, the study is of limited value as evidence of safety because the positive control failed to show an increase in dominant lethal mutations. The Ames mutagenicity test was considered to have been well conducted, and provided no evidence of mutagenicity of irradiated chicken.

The chronic/carcinogenicity study in the mouse seemed to show an increase in testicular tumours, an increase in glomerulonephropathy and decreased survival. However, after thorough review by FDA pathologists and by the Board of Scientific Counsellors of the US National Toxicology Program, which met and discussed its review in public session, it was concluded that the increase in testicular tumours could not be confirmed as treatment-related. In addition, FDA scientists concluded that the increase in glomerulonephropathy and decreased survival in mice were not due to irradiated chicken.

Even though high doses of irradiation were used, the fact that irradiation was carried out at temperatures far below freezing and in the absence of air meant that fewer radiolytic products were formed than when chicken is irradiated unfrozen or in the presence of air. Nevertheless, the lack of treatment-related effects in the many well conducted studies provides additional assurance that the consumption of irradiated food does not pose a hazard.

6.2.3 Human feeding studies in China

In a well designed and carefully controlled double-blind clinical study, 35 different kinds of irradiated food were fed to healthy human volunteers (Anon, 1987; Shao & Feng, 1988). The same diet, but of nonirradiated food, was fed to a control group. The food consisted of grains (two kinds), beans and bean products (10 kinds), vegetables and fruits (more than 20 kinds), meats, fish, eggs and poultry (30 kinds) and flavourings (10 kinds). Meats were irradiated at a dose of 8 kGy, bean products, dried dates, lotus seeds and day lily at a dose of 1–1.5 kGy, and rice, flour, soyabean, red bean, peanut, mushrooms and other fruits and vegetables at less than 1 kGy. The average daily intake of meat was 40 g, of fruits and vegetables, 300 g, and of grain, 470 g, representing irradiation of 60.3% of the total diet.

A total of 70 healthy volunteers (36 male and 34 female medical students) were randomly divided into an irradiated food group and a control group, and tested for 90 days. All were nonsmokers. The caloric and nutrient intakes met the recommended daily values. Complete physical examinations were carried out before and after consumption of irradiated and control foods. Chromosome numerical and structural aberrations, sister chromatid exchange (SCE) and micronuclei in lymphocytes were recorded. An Ames mutagenicity test on urine was also conducted. The subjects were unaware of which type of food they were eating. No adverse effects were seen on activities of daily life, study or physical exercise. Physical examination found no effect of consuming a diet consisting of irradiated foods for 90 days.

No significant differences were seen in either chromatid gaps or breaks, chromosomal fragments, or dicentrics between the group consuming irradiated food and the controls, 100 metaphases being observed per individual. Slight but nonsignificant differences were observed in the frequency of aberrations before feeding irradiated food and after completion of the study, but these were comparable to the differences found in the control group.

There was no statistically significant increase in polyploidy in the group consuming irradiated food compared with the controls; a total of 1000 metaphases per individual were examined so as to give a sample size large enough to enable frequencies below 1% to be measured. For unknown reasons, the frequency of polyploidy was higher in both groups after completion of the study than before (controls: 0.86 ± 0.88 before and 2.86 ± 2.32 after; irradiated food group: 0.66 ± 0.77 before and 3.51 ± 1.95 after). These increases were not treatment-related as they occurred in both irradiated food and control groups.

Lymphocyte micronuclei were examined by concentration and cultivation and no significant differences found. There were no significant findings for SCE.

The 24-hour urine of six volunteers from each group was collected for Ames mutagenicity testing, using strains TA98 and 100 with and without S9 just before the end, and at the end of the study. No differences were seen between controls and treated subjects.

6.2.4 Other studies

In 1987, the FDA announced the filing of a food additive petition proposing the use of a source of gamma radiation to irradiate poultry for the purpose of extending shelf-life and reducing the risk of *Salmonella* contamination (Food and Drug Administration, 1987). Toxicity data were submitted in support of this petition, including a series of three feeding studies carried out at the Central Institute for Nutrition and Food Research (CIVO) in the Netherlands and comprising a multigeneration study in rats, a chronic 2-year study in rats, and a 1-year toxicity study in beagle dogs.

In the multigeneration study, rats were fed a control basal diet, or a diet containing chicken irradiated at 3 or 6 kGy, or nonirradiated chicken (35% of the diet). There were no treatment-related effects for the reproductive parameters measured (fertility, number of pups per litter and post-implantation loss) nor were any treatment-related effects found for body weight, growth rate, or mortality among pups.

A 90-day subchronic feeding study was conducted with animals from the second litter of the third generation. Typical subchronic parameters were measured (body weight, organ weight, haematological parameters, blood and urine chemistry, gross and histological features of organs and tissues). Body weights were slightly increased in the test group, as were relative weights of liver and kidney in the low-dose groups. No gross or histological changes or abnormalities were found. It can be concluded that chicken irradiated at 3 and 6 kGy and fed to rats at a dietary level of 35% over four generations did not cause any deleterious effects.

In the chronic 2-year study, rats were fed either a standard diet or a diet containing nonirradiated or irradiated chicken (3 or 6 kGy) at a level of 35%

dry matter. Each diet was fed to 60 male and 60 female rats. All parameters typical of chronic 2-year rat studies were measured, including behaviour, mortality, growth, haematological parameters, blood and urine chemistry, and gross and histological features of organs and tissues. No differences were found among the groups in appearance, behaviour, mortality or growth. Haematological factors and blood and urine chemistry did not show distinct or consistent changes among groups. No treatment-related effects were found in either the gross or microscopic appearance of organs and tissues.

In the beagle dog study, males and females were fed for 1 year a standard diet or a diet containing 35% of chicken either nonirradiated or irradiated at 3 or 6 kGy. Each group consisted of four males and four females. The health, survival, appearance, behaviour and growth of the animals were not noticeably affected by the inclusion of irradiated chicken in the diet. No evidence of abnormalities in haematological factors, organ weights, or the gross or microscopic appearance of organs and tissues was found.

The CIVO studies provide no evidence of a treatment-related toxicological effect. The only doubtful aspect of the experimental design was the addition of the antioxidant, ethoxyquin, to inhibit rancidity, as it may have confounded interpretation of the study results. However, because ethoxyquin was only added to the chicken meat after irradiation, it was unlikely to have altered the level or kind of radiolytic products formed. Furthermore, the concentration of ethoxyquin was only 35 mg/kg, far less than the levels shown to cause chemical carcinogenesis. Consequently, the FDA was able to conclude that the studies were well conducted and indicated an absence of adverse effects.

6.2.5 International Project in the Field of Food Irradiation

This project was initiated in 1970 to coordinate testing activities. Its headquarters were located at the Federal Research Centre for Nutrition, Karlsruhe, Federal Republic of Germany. All the primary studies under this project are included in the electronic database discussed in section 6.2.1. The project involved a consortium of international agencies and national governments, and the feeding studies contracted by it covered a range of commodities irradiated at dose levels of up to 10 kGy. This dose range was selected because, with the exception of the USA, there was no interest in applications in which such levels of irradiation were exceeded.

During its 12 years (1970–1982) of operation, the project produced 67 technical reports and four activity reports. Two extensive monographs were published (Elias & Cohen, 1977, 1983), together with a report describing a comprehensive programme of *in vivo* mutagenicity testing (Renner et al., 1982). None of the studies gave any indication of the presence of radiation-induced carcinogens or other toxic substances.

6.3 Summary and conclusions

As discussed in Chapter 4, a large number of different chemical compounds are formed in food during irradiation, most of which are already present in the food item in small quantities, or in other food items, or are formed in the course of other forms of treatment, e.g. heating and drying. The macronutrient composition of a particular food is critical in determining what chemical compounds will finally be formed. It would be impossible to perform a toxicological examination and evaluation of each individual component.

A testing programme based on analytical chemistry and experimental toxicology has therefore evolved over the years. Animal studies on irradiated food items and macronutrients, *in vitro* mutagenicity studies on irradiated mixtures and defined chemicals, together with a knowledge of chemical structures and their occurrence and reactivity have provided the basis for the present safety assessments.

The conclusion reached by the Joint FAO/IAEA/WHO Expert Committee on the Wholesomeness of Irradiated Food (WHO, 1980) that the irradiation of any foodstuff at an average radiation dose of up to 10 kGy is toxicologically insignificant and that additional toxicological examinations of such foods are not therefore required has been carefully examined. In the Committee's final evaluation, the general acceptance of a dose of 10 kGy for all types of foods was based on a multitude of animal feeding studies carried out on different classes of food and on the evaluation of the chemical compounds formed by the irradiation of the principal components of food, namely protein, fat and carbohydrates. The Committee also considered studies made available to it on animal colonies reared on irradiated diets, including some on the comparison of diets sterilized by autoclaving or irradiation (25–44 kGy) or treated to destroy pathogens at 15 kGy and multigeneration and carcinogenicity studies; they were performed by institutes in Austria, Denmark, France, Hungary, the Netherlands and the United Kingdom. The Committee concluded that there were no apparent differences between irradiated and nonirradiated diets in studies where the number of animals examined ranged from 5000 to 500 000.

The majority of the toxicological investigations on irradiated foods are concerned with irradiation at doses lower than 10 kGy and most often in the range 0.1–2 kGy. This is both because many foods, e.g. fruit and fish, are unable to tolerate irradiation at higher doses, and because the use of such high doses was found to be unnecessary for the preservation of the food. However, animal studies are available for foods irradiated in the dosage range 10–60 kGy.

With the aim of increasing the sensitivity of the toxicological investigations, a number of short-term *in vivo* and *in vitro* tests have been carried out in an attempt to find unique mutagenic and potentially carcinogenic compounds in irradiated foods and concentrates of such foods.

In studies reviewed again here, there is nothing in the toxicological data to suggest that any of the compounds identified constitute a toxicological risk in the amounts in which they occur in irradiated foods. The data available are qualitatively sufficient for a scientific evaluation of this kind, while on a quantitative basis it is safe to conclude that:

— food irradiation is the most thoroughly investigated food technology from a toxicological point of view;
— different foods of similar composition give rise to similar radiolytic products, thus allowing for extrapolation from one food item to another;
— the toxicological database indicates no adverse toxicological effects of this technology in the radiation dose ranges tested;
— the sensitivity of the toxicology database is adequate because in many of the studies animals were fed diets containing radiolytic products in amounts greater than those expected to be present in human diets.

References[1]

Aiyar AS, Rao S (1977) Studies on mutagenicity of irradiated solutions in *Salmonella typhimurium. Mutation research*, **48**:17–27.

Anon (1976a) To study the toxicological effects of feeding irradiated bananas to rats. *Food irradiation information*, **6** (Suppl.):109.

Anon (1976b) To investigate the wholesomeness of irradiated bananas fed to dogs. *Food irradiation information*, **6** (Suppl.):107.

Anon (1980) *A study of possible mutagenicity of irradiated onion powder by Salmonella/mammalian-microsome mutagenicity tests.* Karlsruhe, Federal Research Centre for Nutrition (IFIP Technical Report).

Anon (1987) Safety evaluation of 35 kinds of irradiated human foods. *Chinese medical journal*, **100**(9):715–718.

Anukaranhanonta T et al. (1980) *Wholesomeness study of irradiated salted and dried mackerel in rats.* Vienna, International Atomic Energy Agency (Summarized Technical Report, IAEA contract 1609/RB and 1609/R1/RB).

Anukaranhanonta T et al. (1981) Wholesomeness study of irradiated salted and dried mackerel in rats. In: *Wholesomeness of the process of food irradiation.* Vienna, International Atomic Energy Agency (IAEA Technical Document, No. 256), pp. 7–42.

---

[1] Except where otherwise indicated, unpublished documents included in this listing can be obtained by writing to Food and Drug Administration, Dockets Management Branch, Park Building, Rockville, MD, USA, mentioning FDA docket nos. 81N-0004, 86F-0507 and 86F-0509.

Aravindakshan M, Sundaram K (1978) Studies on the safety evaluation of radurized Indian mackerel. In: *Food preservation by irradiation*, Vol. II. Vienna, International Atomic Energy Agency, pp. 53–61.

Aravindakshan M et al. (1978) Multigeneration feeding studies with an irradiated whole diet. In: *Food preservation by irradiation*, Vol. II. Vienna, International Atomic Energy Agency, pp. 41–51.

Aravindakshan M et al. (1980a) *Ninety-day feeding and reproduction study on irradiated onion in rats*. Karlsruhe, Federal Research Centre for Nutrition (IFIP Technical Report IFIP-R59).

Aravindakshan M et al. (1980b) *Mutagenicity evaluation of irradiated onion in the germ cell of male mouse as revealed by the dominant lethal test*. Pre-print of work on contract IFIP 1612/R3/CF.

Armendares S et al. (1971) Chromosome abnormalities in severe protein calorie malnutrition. *Nature*, **232**:271.

Baev I (1980) *Investigation of wholesomeness of feeding low-irradiated diet to mice*. Vienna, International Atomic Energy Agency (IAEA Report No. R-2036/F).

Baev I et al. (1981) *Investigation of wholesomeness studies of feeding irradiated diet to mice*. Vienna, International Atomic Energy Agency (IAEA Technical Report No. 256).

Bernardes B (1980) *Short-term toxicity studies of irradiated coffee and black beans*. Karlsruhe, Federal Research Centre for Nutrition (IFIP Technical Report).

Bernardes B et al. (1981) Short-term toxicity studies of irradiated black beans (*P. vulgaris*). In: *Wholesomeness of the process of food irradiation*. Vienna, International Atomic Energy Agency (IAEA Technical Document No. 256), pp. 67–80.

Bhaskaram C, Sadasivan G (1975) Effects of feeding irradiated wheat to malnourished children. *American journal of nutrition*, **28**:130–135.

Biagini C et al. (1967) Growth and fertility of mice fed an irradiated diet for two years. *Giornale de medicina militare*, **117**:347–368.

Blood FR et al. (1966) Feeding of irradiated chicken, beef and pineapple jam to dogs. *Toxicology and applied pharmacology*, **8**:241–246.

Bone JF (1963) *The growth, breeding, longevity and histopathology of rats fed irradiated or control foods (histopathological studies)*. US Army, unpublished contract report no. DA-49-193-MD-2064.

Bradley MV et al. (1968) Low pH of irradiated sucrose in induction of chromosome aberrations. *Nature*, **217**:1182–1183.

Bradsky W, Vryvaeva IV (1977) Cell polyploidy: its relation to tissue growth and function. *International review of cytology*, **50**:275–332.

Brin M et al. (1961a) Effects of feeding X-irradiated pork to rats on their pyridoxine nutrition as reflected in the activity of plasma transaminase. *Journal of nutrition*, **75**:35–38.

Brin M et al. (1961b) Effects of feeding X-irradiated pork to rats on their thiamine nutrition as reflected in the activity of erythrocyte transketolase. *Journal of nutrition*, **75**:29–34.

Brin M et al. (1961c) The effects of feeding irradiated pork, bread, green beans and shrimp to rats on growth and on five enzymes in blood. *Toxicology and applied pharmacology*, **3**:606–617.

Bronnikova IA, Okuneva LA (1973) Research on the mutagenic and cytotoxic properties of irradiated foodstuffs. *Voprosy pitanija*, **32** (4): 46–50 (translation from Russian; FDA docket no. 81N-0004).

Brownell LE et al. (1959) *Growth, reproduction, mortality and pathologic changes in rats fed gamma-irradiated potatoes.* US Army, unpublished contract report no. DA-49-007-MD-581.

Bubl EC (1961) *Short and long-term survival and breeding capacity of rats fed high levels of foodstuffs sterilized by ionizing radiation (ground pork).* US Army, unpublished contract report no. DA-49-007-MD-580.

Bugyaki L (1973) To study the effect of feeding irradiated wheat flour to mice. *Food irradiation information,* **2** (Suppl.):vii.

Bugyaki L et al. (1964) Do irradiated foodstuffs have a radiomimetic effect? II. Trials with mice fed wheat meal irradiated at 5 Mrad. *Atompraxis*, **14**:112.

Burns GH, Abrams GD (1961) *Necrotizing arteritis in rats used in a toxicity study of irradiated potatoes.* US Army, unpublished contract report, no. DA-49-007-MD-581.

Chaubey RC et al. (1978) Mutagenicity evaluation of irradiated Indian mackerel in Swiss mice. In: *Food preservation by irradiation*, Vol. II. Vienna, International Atomic Energy Agency.

Chauhan PS et al. (1975a) Studies on dominant lethal mutations in third generation rats reared on an irradiated diet. *International journal of radiation biology*, **28**:215–223.

Chauhan PS et al. (1975b) Dominant lethal mutations in male mice fed gamma-irradiated diet. *Food and cosmetic toxicology*, **13**:433–436.

Chauhan PS et al (1977) Evaluation of freshly irradiated wheat for dominant lethal mutations in Wistar rats. *Toxicology*, **7**:85–97.

Chopra VL (1965) Tests on *Drosophila* for the production of mutations by irradiated medium or irradiated DNA. *Nature*, **208**:609–700.

Chopra VL et al. (1963) Cytological effects observed in plant material grown on irradiated fruit juices. *Radiation botany*, **3**:1–6.

Clarkson TB, Pick JR (1964) *The effect of control ground beef and irradiated 5.58 Mrad ground beef consumption on reproduction. Final report*. Washington, DC, US Surgeon General's Office (Contract No. DA-49-193-MD-2098).

Coquet B et al. (1980) *Irradiated legumes; toxicity and reproduction studies in the rat*. Karlsruhe, Federal Research Centre for Nutrition (IFIP Technical Report).

Dahlgren RR et al. (1977) *Hamster teratology study. Final report*. US Army, unpublished contract report no. DAMD-17-76-C-6047.

Dahlgren RR et al. (1980) *Animal feeding studies of irradiated sterilized chicken*. Karlsruhe, Federal Research Centre for Nutrition (IFIP Thirteenth Quarterly Report).

de Knecht-van Echelen A et al. (1971) *Multi-generation study in rats with radiation-pasteurized chicken*. Zeist, Central Institute for Nutrition and Food Research (IFIP Technical Report No. R3622).

de Knecht-van Echelen A et al. (1972) *Chronic (two-year) feeding study in rats with radiation-pasteurized chicken*. Zeist, Central Institute for Nutrition and Food Research (IFIP Technical Report No. R3773).

den Drijver L et al. (1986) High-performance liquid chromatographic determination of D-arabino-hexos-2-ulose (D-glucosone) in irradiated sugar solutions. Application of the method to irradiated mango. *Journal of agricultural and food chemistry*, **34**:758–762.

Dent NJ et al. (1977) *An investigation of the elevated serum alkaline phosphatase levels in rats fed irradiated fish diets*. Karlsruhe, Federal Research Centre for Nutrition (IFIP Technical Report, IFIP-R42).

Derse PH (1978) *Dominant lethal studies on rats fed a diet containing 15% Kent mangoes. Final report*. Karlsruhe, Federal Research Centre for Nutrition (IFIP Technical Report WARF-T-606).

Derse PH (1979) *Chromosome aberration study, F1 generation. Final report.* Karlsruhe, Federal Research Centre for Nutrition.

Dixon MS et al. (1961) Influence of irradiated bacon lipids on body growth, incidence of cancer, and other pathologic changes in mice. *Journal of food science,* **26**:611–617.

Elias PS, Cohen AJ, eds. (1977) *Radiation chemistry of major food components,* Amsterdam, Elsevier.

Elias PS, Cohen AJ, eds. (1983) *Recent advances in food irradiation.* Amsterdam, Elsevier Biomedical.

Eriksen WH, Emborg C (1972) The effect on pre-implantation death of feeding rats on radiation-sterilized food. *International journal of radiation biology,* **22**(3): 131–135.

Farkas J et al. (1981) Evaluation of possible mutagenicity of irradiated spices. *Acta alimentaria,* **10**:129–135.

Fegley HC, Edmonds RE (1976) To examine the wholesomeness of irradiated soft-shell clams (*Mya arenaria*) in dogs. *Food irradiation information,* **6** (Suppl.):111.

Food and Drug Administration (1982) *Toxicological principles for the safety assessments of direct food additives and color additives used in food.* Rockville, MD.

Food and Drug Administration (1986) *Federal register,* **51**:13376–13399.

Food and Drug Administration (1987) *Federal register,* **52**:6391.

Frohberg H, Schulze-Schencking MS (1975) *In vivo* cytogenetic investigation in bone-marrow of rats, Chinese hamsters and mice treated with 6-mercaptopurine. *Archives of toxicology,* **33**:209–224.

Gabriel KL, Edmonds RS (1976a) To study the effects of radurized onions when fed to beagle dogs. *Food irradiation information,* **6** (Suppl.):116.

Gabriel KL, Edmonds RS (1976b) To study the effects of radurized onions when fed to albino rats. *Food irradiation information,* **6** (Suppl.):118.

Gabriel KL, Edmonds RS (1977a) To study the effects of radurized sweet cherries, apricots and prune-plums when fed to albino rats. *Food irradiation information,* **7** (Suppl.):138.

Gabriel KL, Edmonds RS (1977b) To study the effects of radurized sweet cherries, apricots, and prune-plums when fed to dogs. *Food irradiation information,* **7** (Suppl.):140.

George KP et al. (1976) Frequency of polyploid cells in the bone marrow of rats fed irradiated wheat. *Food and cosmetic toxicology*, **14**(4):289–291.

Hale MW et al. (1960) *Growth, reproduction, mortality and pathologic changes in dogs fed gamma-irradiated bacon for two years*. US Army, unpublished final contract report no. DA-49-007-MD-780.

Hattori Y et al. (1979) Mutagenicity tests of irradiated onions by *Escherichia coli* mutants *in vitro*. *Mutation research*, **60**:115–119.

Hickman JR (1975a) To establish the toxicological safety of skin-on cod fillets that have been irradiated in order to extend the chilled (0–4 °C) storage life when fed to rats. *Food irradiation information*, **5** (Suppl.):96.

Hickman JR (1975b) To obtain data in support of the use of radiation for the elimination of salmonellae from frozen horse meat. *Food irradiation information*, **5** (Suppl.):91.

Hickman JR et al. (1964) Rat feeding studies on wheat treated with gamma radiation. I. Reproduction. *Food and cosmetic toxicology*, **2**:15–21.

Hickman JR et al. (1969a) *Studies on the wholesomeness of irradiated fish. Reproduction*. Harwell, UK Atomic Energy Authority (Technical Report AERE-R-6016).

Hickman JR et al. (1969b) *Studies on the wholesomeness of irradiated fish. 90-day toxicity test*. Harwell, UK Atomic Energy Authority (Technical Report AERE-R-R-6017).

Hickman JR et al. (1969c) *Studies on the wholesomeness of irradiated fish. Growth, survival and pathology*. Harwell, UK Atomic Energy Authority (Technical Report, AERE-R-6015).

Hilliard WG (1974) To provide clinical, haematological and pathological observations during an 18-month trial of feeding onion-incorporated diets, whether irradiated or non-irradiated, to dogs for determination of any imparted toxicity. *Food irradiation information*, **3** (Suppl.):24.

Hilliard WG et al. (1966) Long-term effects of feeding irradiated onion to dogs. *Food and cosmetic toxicology*, **4**:557.

Hofer H et al. (1979) *Cytogenetic investigations on the effect of irradiated foods*. Karlsruhe, Federal Research Centre for Nutrition (final report to IFIP).

Hossain M (1979) *Studies on the safety and wholesomeness of irradiated fish*. Vienna, International Atomic Energy Agency (IAEA Contract No. 1919 RB).

Hossain MM et al. (1981) Studies on wholesomeness of irradiated shrimp and carp. In: *Wholesomeness of the process of food irradiation.* Vienna, International Atomic Energy Agency (IAEA Technical Document No. 265), pp. 43–65.

Huntingdon Research Centre (1975) *Reproduction and longevity of rats fed an irradiated potato diet.* Karlsruhe, International Project in the Field of Food Irradiation, Institut für Strahlentechnologie (IFIP Technical Report IFIP-R25).

Huntingdon Research Centre (1978) *1. Multigeneration reproduction study. 2. Mutagenicity study. 3. Teratology study.* Karlsruhe, International Project in the Field of Food Irradiation, Institut für Strahlentechnologie (IFIP Technical Report IFIP-R49).

Huntingdon Research Centre (1979) *Studies in mice fed a diet containing irradiated fish. Eighty-week feeding study.* Karlsruhe, International Project in the Field of Food Irradiation, Institut für Strahlentechnologie (IFIP Technical Report IFIP-R50).

Ikeda Y et al. (1969) Study on the safety of g-irradiated wheat. Chronic toxicity test in the rat. Long term toxicity study of irradiated wheat in the rat. (Tables only, FDA docket no. 81N-0004).

Ikeda Y (1971) *Safety studies on g-irradiated potatoes.* Final Report on the Preservation of Potatoes by Irradiation. Addendum (translation from Japanese).

Inveresk Research International (1976) *90-day toxicity and reproductive toxicity of irradiated European plaice (Pleuronectes platessa).* Karlsruhe, International Project in the Field of Food Irradiation, Institut für Strahlentechnologie (IFIP Technical Report IFIP-R41).

Jaarma M, Henricson B (1964) On the wholesomeness of gamma irradiated potatoes. *Acta veterinaria scandinavica*, **5**:238.

Jaarma M, Bengtsson G (1966) On the wholesomeness of gamma-irradiated potatoes. II. Feeding experiments with pigs. *Nutritio et dieta*, **8**:109.

Jaarma M et al. (1966) On the wholesomeness of gamma-irradiated potatoes. III. Feeding experiments with rats. *Nutritio et dieta*, **8**:296.

Joner PE et al. (1978) Mutagenicity testing of irradiated cod fillets. *Lebensmittel-Wissenschaft und Technologie,* **11**:224–226.

Kesavan PC, Swaminathan MS (1966) Cytotoxic and radiomimetic activity of irradiated culture medium on human leukocytes. *Current science*, **35**(16):403–404.

Khan AH, Alderson T (1965) Mutagenic effect of irradiated and unirradiated DNA in *Drosophila. Nature*, **208**:700–702.

Leonard A et al. (1977) Mutagenicity tests with irradiated food in the mouse. *Strahlentherapie*, **153**:349–351.

Levinsky HV, Wilson MA (1975) Mutagenic evaluation of an alcoholic extract from gamma-irradiated potatoes. *Food and cosmetic toxicology*, **13**:243–246.

Levinsky HV, Wilson M, MacFarland HN (1973) *A study of the mutagenic effects of an alcoholic extract of irradiated potatoes in the mouse*. Karlsruhe, International Project in the Field of Food Irradiation, Institut für Strahlentechnologie (IFIP Technical Report IFIP-R9).

Loaharanu SP (1978) Feeding studies of irradiated foods with insects. In: *Food preservation by irradiation*, Vol. II, Vienna, International Atomic Energy Agency, pp. 113-131.

Loosli JK et al. (1964) *Components of ionized irradiated meats injurious to reproduction. Final report.* Washington, DC, Office of Surgeon General (US Army, contract no. DA49-193-MD-2097).

Lorand Eötvös University of Sciences and Central Food Research Institute (1979) *Teratogenic studies on albino rats fed diets containing either irradiated ground pepper, mild paprika or spice mixture*. Karlsruhe, International Project in the Field of Food Irradiation, Institut für Strahlentechnologie (IFIP Technical Report IFIP-R52).

Luckey TD et al. (1973) Apollo diet evaluation: a comparison of biological and analytical methods including bioisolation of mice and gamma-irradiation of diet. *Aerospace medicine*, **44**:888–901.

Lusskin RM (1979) *Evaluation of the mutagenicity of irradiated sterilized chicken by the sex-linked recessive lethal test in Drosophila melanogaster*. Contract Final Report (FDA docket no. 84F-0230).

Malhotra OP, Reber EF (1963a) Effect of methionine and age of rats on the occurrence of hemorrhagic diathesis in rats fed a ration containing irradiated beef. *Journal of nutrition*, **80**:85–90.

Malhotra OP, Reber EF (1963b) Methionine and testosterone affect occurrence of hemorrhagic diathesis in rats. *American journal of physiology*, **205**:1089–1092.

Malhotra OP et al. (1965) Effect of methionine and vitamin K3 on hemorrhages induced by feeding a ration containing irradiated beef. *Toxicology and applied pharmacology*, **7**:402–408.

McCay CM, Rumsey GL (1961) *Effect of ionizing radiation on the nutritive value of potatoes as determined by growth, reproduction and lactation studies with dogs*. Department of the Army, unpublished contract report DA-49-007-MD-600.

McGown EL et al. (1979) *Investigation of possible antithiamin properties in irradiation sterilized chicken.* US Army, unpublished final contract report D6-47.

McKee RW et al. (1959) *The influence of irradiated lipids on the incidence of spontaneous mammary carcinoma and hepatoma in strains A/HE and C3H mice.* US Army, unpublished final contract report, DA-49-007-MD-579.

Metwalli OM (1977) Study on the effect of food irradiation on some blood serum enzymes in rats. *Zeitschrift für Ernährungswissenschaft,* **16**:18–21.

Mittler S (1979) Failure of irradiated beef and ham to induce genetic aberrations in *Drosophila. International journal of radiation biology,* **35**:583–588.

Mittler S (1980) *Mutagenicity evaluation of irradiated onion powder.* Progress Report to McCormick & Co. Inc. (FDA docket no. 84F-0230).

Mittler S, Eiss MI (1982) Failure of irradiated onion powder to induce sex-linked recessive lethal mutations in *Drosophila melanogaster. Mutation research,* **104**:113.

Monsen H (1960) Heart lesions in mice induced by feeding irradiated foods. *Federation proceedings,* **19**:1031–1034.

Moran ET et al. (1968) Effect of cobalt-60 gamma irradiation on the utilization of energy, protein, and phosphorus from wheat bran by the chicken. *Cereal chemistry,* **45**:469–479.

Moutschen-Dahmen M et al. (1970) Pre-implantation death of mouse eggs caused by irradiated food. *International journal of radiation biology,* **18**:201–216.

Münzner R, Renner HW (1975) [Mutagenicity testing of irradiated laboratory animal diet by the host mediated assay with *S. typhimurium* G46.] *International journal of radiation biology,* **27**:371–375 (in German).

Münzner R, Renner HW (1981) Mutagenicity testing of irradiated onion powder. *Journal of food science,* **46**:1269–1270.

Nadkarni GB (1980) *Wholesomeness studies in rats fed irradiated Indian mackerel.* Karlsruhe, International Project in the Field of Food Irradiation, Federal Research Centre for Nutrition (IFIP Technical Report R-54).

Nees PO (1970) *Chronic toxicity studies on irradiated strawberries. Rat study. Vol. 2.* Contract Report to Atomic Energy of Canada (AEC Contract no. AT-(11-1)-1722).

Nees PO, Sharma RN (1970) *Chronic toxicity studies on irradiated strawberries. Dog studies. Vol. 1.* Contract Report to Atomic Energy of Canada (AEC Contract no. AT(11-1)-1722).

Osipova IN (1974) [Investigation of the possible mutagenicity of extracts from irradiated potatoes as a function of storage and cooking.] *Voprosy pitanija*, **33**(1):78–81 (in Russian).

Osipova IN et al. (1975) [Influence of the storage and culinary treatment of irradiated potatoes on the cytogenetic activity of potato extracts.] *Voprosy pitanija*, **34**(4):54–57 (in Russian).

Palmer AK et al. (1973) *Reproduction and longevity of rats fed an irradiated potato diet: 4th interim report—dominant lethal assay and cytogenetics.* Interim Report of International Project in the Field of Food Irradiation, unpublished.

Paynter OE (1959) *Long-term feeding and reproduction studies on irradiated corn and tuna.* US Army, unpublished contract report no. DA-49-007-MD-788.

Phillips AW et al. (1961a) *Long-term rat feeding studies: irradiated chicken stew and cabbage.* US Army unpublished contract report no. DA-49-007-MD-783.

Phillips AW et al. (1961b) *Long-term feeding studies: irradiated oranges.* Final contract report, US Army contract no. DA-49-007-MD-791.

Porter G, Festing M (1970) A comparison between irradiated and autoclaved diets for breeding mice with observations on palatability. *Laboratory animals*, **4**:203–213.

Proctor BG (1971) *A study of the carcinogenicity of irradiated chicken in the mouse.* Technical Report to the AEC, Canada, Project 245.

Proctor BG (1974) To determine the presence of carcinogenic substances in irradiated chicken by oral administration of the test food to mice throughout their entire life span. *Food irradiation information*, **3** (Suppl.):18.

Radomski JL et al. (1965a) A study of the possible carcinogenicity of irradiated foods. *Toxicology and applied pharmacology*, **7**:122–127.

Radomski JL et al. (1965b) Chronic toxicity studies on irradiated beef stew and evaporated milk. *Toxicology and applied pharmacology*, **7**:113–121.

Raltech Scientific Services (1979) *Toxicology studies on rats fed a diet containing 15% irradiated Kent mangoes.* Karlsruhe, International Project in the Field of Food Irradiation, Institut für Strahlentechnologie (IFIP Technical Report IFIP-R51).

Raltech Scientific Services (1981) *Toxicology studies in rats fed a diet containing 15% irradiated Kent mangoes. Two-year feeding study.* Karlsruhe, International Project in the Field of Food Irradiation, Federal Research Centre for Nutrition (IFIP Technical Report IFIP-R58).

Raltech Scientific Services (1982) *Irradiated sterilized chicken meat: a chronic toxicity and reproductive performance study in beagle dogs.* Unpublished document (FDA docket no. 84F-0230).

Raltech Scientific Services (1983) *Mouse bioassay of irradiated chicken.* (Unpublished document; available on microfiche from National Technical Information Service, 5285 Port Royal Road, Springfield, VA 22161, USA).

Read MS, Kraybill HF (1958) Short-term rat feeding studies with gamma-irradiated food products. *Journal of nutrition*, **65**:39–51.

Read MS et al. (1961) Successive generation rat feeding studies with a composite diet of gamma-irradiated foods. *Toxicology and applied pharmacology*, **3**:153–173.

Reber EF et al. (1959) The effects of feeding irradiated flour to dogs. I. Growth. *Toxicology*, **1**:55–60.

Reber EF et al. (1960) The effects of feeding irradiated beef to dogs. I. Growth. *American journal of veterinary research*, **21**:367–370.

Reber EF et al. (1961) The effects of feeding irradiated flour to dogs. II. Reproduction and pathology. *Toxicology and applied pharmacology*, **3**:568–573.

Reber EF et al. (1962) The effects of feeding irradiated beef to dogs. II. Reproduction and pathology. *American journal of veterinary research*, **23**:74–76.

Reddi OS et al. (1972) Effect of irradiated wheat on germ cells in mice. *Indian journal of medical research*, **60**:1543–1546.

Reddi OS et al. (1977) Lack of genetic and cytogenetic effects in mice fed on irradiated wheat. *International journal of radiation biology*, **34**:589–601.

Renner HW (1977) Chromosome studies on bone marrow cells of Chinese hamsters fed a radiosterilized diet. *Toxicology*, **8**:213–222.

Renner HW, Reichelt D (1973) Safety of high concentrations of free radicals in irradiated foodstuffs. *Zentralblatt für Veterinärmedizin, Reihe B*, **20**:648–660.

Renner HW et al. (1973) Mutagenicity of irradiated foodstuffs with the dominant lethal test. *Humangenetik*, **18**(2):155–164.

Renner HW et al. (1982) An investigation of the genetic toxicology of irradiated foodstuffs using short-term test systems. Part 3. *In vivo* tests in small rodents and in *Drosophila melanogaster. Food and chemical toxicology*, **20**:867–876.

Richardson LR (1960) *A long-term feeding study of irradiated chicken and green beans using the rat as the experimental animal.* US Army, unpublished contract report no. DA-49-007-MD-582.

Rinehart RR, Ratty FJ (1965) Mutation in *Drosophila melanogaster* cultured on irradiated food. *Genetics,* **52**(6):1119–1126.

Rinehart RR, Ratty FJ (1967) Mutation in *Drosophila melanogaster* cultured on irradiated whole food or food components. *International journal of radiation biology,* **12**:347–354.

Ronning DC (1980) *Animal feeding studies protocol for irradiated sterilized chicken. Final Report: Dominant lethal study.* US Army, unpublished contract report no. DAMD 17-76-C-6047.

Ross ST et al. (1970) Cytological effects of juice or puree from irradiated strawberries. *Journal of food science,* **35**:549–550.

Schlatter C et al. (1980) *Drosophila mutagenicity tests with irradiated dates.* Karlsruhe, Federal Research Centre for Nutrition (Technical Report).

Schubert J et al. (1967) Hydroxyalkyl peroxides and the toxicity of irradiated sucrose. *International journal of radiation biology,* **13**(5):485–489.

Schubert J et al. (1973) Irradiated strawberries — chemical cytogenetic and antibacterial properties. *Journal of agricultural and food chemistry,* **21**(4): 684–692.

Shao S, Feng J (1988) [Safety estimation of persons feeding from 35 kinds of irradiated diets — chromosome aberrations and SCE analysis of cultured lymphocyte.] *Journal of Chinese radiation medicine and protection,* **3**:271 (in Chinese).

Shaw MW, Hayes E (1966) Effects of irradiated sucrose on the chromosomes of human lymphocytes *in vitro. Nature,* **211**:1254–1257.

Shillinger YI, Kamaldinova ZN (1973) [The wholesomeness of potatoes irradiated with an accelerated electron beam and gamma-irradiation for the purpose of inhibiting sprouting.] *Voprosy pitanija,* **32**(6):50–55 (in Russian).

Shillinger I, Osipova IN (1970) [The effect of fresh fish, exposed to gamma radiation on the organism of albino rats.] *Voprosy pitanija,* **29**(5):45–50 (in Russian).

Swaminathan MS et al. (1962) Cytological aberrations observed in barley embryos cultured in irradiated potato mash. *Radiation research,* **16**:182–188.

Swaminathan MS et al. (1963) *Drosophila melanogaster* reared on irradiated medium. *Science,* **141**:637–638.

Takyi EEK, Ofori-Mensah N (1979) Short-term toxicity study of irradiated cocoa beans in rats. *Journal of the science of food and agriculture,* **32**: 933–940.

Teply LJ, Kline BE (1959) *Possible carcinogenicity of irradiated foods.* US Army, unpublished contract report no. DA-49-007-MD-583 (located in Food Additive Petition 7M 2056, Vol. 9, p. 2150).

Tesh JM, Davidson EJ (1976) *Irradiated wheat: study of its dominant lethal action in the rat.* IFIP Technical Report LSR 76/IF12/158.

Tesh JM, Palmer AK (1980) To investigate the effects of feeding an irradiated wheat flour diet on the incidence of polyploidy and micronucleated polychromatic erythrocytes in bone marrow cells of rats and to assess mutagenic potential by means of the dominant lethal assay. *Food irradiation information,* **10** (Suppl.): 183–184.

Thayer DW et al. (1987) Toxicology studies of irradiated-sterilized chicken. *Journal of food protection,* **50**: 278–288.

Thompson SW et al. (1963) *Histopathology of mice fed irradiated foods.* Technical Report no. 279, Project 3:012501-A-803 (FDA docket no. 84F-0230).

Thomson GM et al. (1977) *Mouse teratology study.* US Army unpublished contract report no. DAMD-17-76-C-6047.

Til HP et al. (1971) *One-year feeding study with low-dose irradiated chicken in beagle dogs.* Zeist, Central Institute for Nutrition and Food Research (report no. R3443).

Tobe M et al. (1980) *Studies on wholesomeness of irradiated rice. A chronic toxicology study with monkeys* (FDA docket no. 84F-0230).

Truhaut R, Saint-Lèbe L (1978) Different approaches to toxicological evaluation of irradiated starch. In: *Food preservation by irradiation,* Vol II. Vienna, International Atomic Energy Agency, pp. 31–39.

Vakil UK (1975a) To study the wholesomeness of feeding gamma-irradiated Red winter wheat flour to mice. *Food irradiation information,* **4** (Suppl.):55.

Vakil UK (1975b) To study the wholesomeness of feeding dehydro-irradiated shrimps to rats. *Food irradiation information,* **4** (Suppl.):49.

Vakil UK (1975c) Wholesomeness of feeding gamma-irradiated red winter wheat to rats (chronic study). *Food irradiation information,* **4** (Suppl.):53.

van Kooij JG, Leveling HB, Schubert J (1978) Application of the Ames mutagenicity test to food processed by physical preservation methods. In: *Food preservation by irradiation,* Vol. II. Vienna, International Atomic Energy Agency, pp. 63–71.

van Logten MJ et al. (1971) The wholesomeness of irradiated mushrooms. *Food and cosmetic toxicology*, **9**:379–388.

van Logten MJ et al. (1972) The wholesomeness of irradiated shrimp. *Food and cosmetic toxicology*, **10**:781–788.

van Logten MJ et al. (1978) *Investigation of the wholesomeness of autoclaved or irradiated food in rats*. Bilthoven, National Institute of Public Health (Report No. 33/78).

van Logten MJ et al. (1983) *Long-term wholesomeness study of autoclaved or irradiated pork in rats*. Bilthoven, National Institute of Public Health (Report no. 17401 001).

van Petten GR et al. (1966) Effect of feeding irradiated onion to consecutive generations of the rat. *Food and cosmetic toxicology*, **4**:593–599.

Varma MB et al. (1986) Lack of clastogenic effects of irradiated glucose in somatic and germ cells of mice. *Mutation research*, **169**:55–59.

Verschuuren HG et al. (1966) Ninety-day rat feeding study on irradiated strawberries. *Food irradiation*, 7(1–2):A17–A21.

Vijayalaxmi (1975) Cytogenetic studies in rats fed irradiated wheat. *International journal of radiation biology*, **27**:283–285.

Vijayalaxmi (1976) Genetic effects of feeding irradiated wheat to mice. *Canadian journal of genetics and cytology*, **18**:231–238.

Vijayalaxmi (1978) Cytogenetic studies in monkeys fed irradiated wheat. *Toxicology*, **9**:181–184.

Vijayalaxmi, Rao KV (1976) Dominant lethal mutations in rats fed on irradiated wheat. *International journal of radiation biology*, **29**:93–98.

Vijayalaxmi, Sadasivan G (1975) Chromosomal aberrations in rats fed irradiated wheat *International journal of radiation biology*, **27**:135–142.

Vlielander L, Chappel C (1968a) *One-year wholesomeness study of irradiated and non-irradiated mushrooms in the rat*. Contract Report to Atomic Energy of Canada, Project 6632, Report no. 2.

Vlielander L, Chappel C (1968b) *One-year wholesomeness study of irradiated and non-irradiated mushrooms in dogs*. Technical Report to Atomic Energy of Canada, Project no. 6632.

Wasserman RH, Trum BF (1955) Effect of feeding dogs the flesh of lethally irradiated cows and sheep. *Science*, **121**:894–896.

WHO (1987) *Principles for the safety assessment of food additives and contaminants in food.* Geneva, World Health Organization (Environmental Health Criteria No. 70).

Wills ED (1981) *Studies of irradiated food.* Karlsruhe, Federal Research Centre for Nutrition (IFIP Technical Report).

Wilmer J et al. (1981) Mutagenicity of gamma-irradiated oxygenated and deoxygenated solutions of 2-deoxy-D-ribose and D-ribose in *Salmonella typhimurium. Mutation research*, 90:385.

Zaitsev AP (1980) *Report on the study of toxicity and mutagenicity of irradiated food products used in an experiment.* Report to the Academy of Medical Sciences, Moscow (FDA docket no. 84F-0230).

Zaitsev AP et al. (1977) Experimental studies of irradiated fish safety. In: *Abstracts, XIV Pacific Science Congress* at Khabaroush, USSR.

Zajcev AN et al. (1975) Toxicologic and hygienic investigation of potatoes irradiated with a beam of fast electrons and gamma rays to control sprouting. *Toxicology*, 4:267–274.

7.
Microbiology

7.1 Introduction

Food is generally irradiated at doses of less than 10 kGy, which are not sufficient to kill all microorganisms that might be present in it. However, irradiation typically results in a massive reduction in the number and variety of microorganisms; for example, Table 14 lists the values of D_{10} for a group of foodborne pathogens in ground beef, fish, oysters, shrimps and liquid whole eggs (D_{10} is defined as the dose of irradiation needed to produce a 10-fold reduction in the population of microorganisms). As can be seen, doses far below 10 kGy result in extensive destruction of common foodborne pathogens in typical foods. Consequently, doses between 1 and 10 kGy can be used in certain instances for the virtual elimination of foodborne pathogens.

The aim of irradiation from the microbiological point of view is to reduce or eliminate spoilage organisms and pathogenic organisms present in food

Table 14. D_{10} values of selected nonsporogenic bacteria

Bacterium	Medium	D_{10} (kGy)	Reference
Vibrio parahaemolyticus	Fish[a]	0.03–0.06	Matches & Liston (1971)
Pseudomonas fluorescens	Ground beef [a]	0.12	Maxcy & Tiwari (1973)
Campylobacter jejuni	Ground beef [a]	0.14–0.16	Tarkowski et al. (1984)
Aeromonas hydrophila	Ground beef [b]	0.14–0.19	Palumbo et al. (1986)
Proteus vulgaris	Oysters[c]	0.20	Quinn et al. (1967)
Yersinia enterocolitica	Ground beef [a]	0.1–0.21	Tarkowski et al. (1984)
Shigella dysenteriae	Shrimp[d]	0.22	Mossel & Stegeman (1985)
Shigella flexneri	Shrimp[d]	0.41	Mossel & Stegeman (1985)
Brucella abortus	Ground beef [a]	0.34	Maxcy & Tiwari (1973)
Escherichia coli	Ground beef [a]	0.43	Maxcy & Tiwari (1973)
Salmonella anatum	Ground beef [a]	0.67	Tarkowski et al. (1984)
Salmonella enteritidis	Ground beef [a]	0.70	Maxcy & Tiwari (1973)
Salmonella newport	Liquid whole egg[e]	0.32	Licciardello et al. (1968)

[a] Irradiated at ambient temperature.
[b] Irradiated at 2°C.
[c] Irradiated at 5°C.
[d] Irradiated frozen.
[e] Irradiated at 0°C.
Adapted from Diehl (1990).

(see Chapter 3). The shelf-life for a given food is therefore extended by irradiation, and illness caused by pathogenic organisms reduced or eliminated. This is of great public health importance as foodborne illness due to microbial contamination is a major health problem in almost all countries (Käferstein, 1990).

7.2 Selective killing and differential growth

Despite the obvious potential value of food irradiation for making food safer, concerns have been expressed about possible hazards arising from its use (Murray, 1990), including the theoretical possibility that normal spoilage organisms may be preferentially destroyed by irradiation, thereby allowing pathogenic organisms to survive and grow unchecked. In the absence of the spoilage organisms, the food would then appear fit for consumption, based on typical organoleptic properties, yet contain increased numbers of pathogens. It is necessary, therefore, to conduct studies on the effect of irradiation on the numbers and types of microorganisms in food immediately following treatment and under the conditions that might prevail in commerce and in the consumer's home (Diehl, 1990). Such studies are an integral part of food technology and are required for establishing the safe use of such traditional nonsterilizing processes as pasteurization, vacuum packing, salting, smoking or other forms of preservation (Advisory Committee on Irradiated and Novel Foods, 1986).

The FDA has recently approved a proposal to irradiate chicken at a maximum dose of 3 kGy to control foodborne pathogens such as *Salmonella, Yersinia* and *Campylobacter* (Anon., 1990). At such doses, the only pathogens likely to survive will be spore-forming organisms (Mulder, 1982). Thus *Clostridium botulinum*, which produces a toxin that can cause illness and death, poses a real problem of microbiological safety because its spores are more resistant than vegetative forms to irradiation (Diehl, 1990; Anon., 1990).

While the FDA recognizes (Anon., 1990) that *Clostridium botulinum* does not ordinarily grow and produce toxin in poultry stored at refrigeration temperatures, it nevertheless considered the theoretical possibility that it could do so without any sign of spoilage obvious to the consumer if the poultry were exposed to higher temperatures. Consequently, the FDA required studies to demonstrate that chicken irradiated at 3 kGy did not pose an increased risk of foodborne disease from *Clostridium botulinum*.

In one series of studies (Firstenberg-Eden et al., 1983; Rowley et al., 1983), chicken skins were inoculated with *Clostridium botulinum* type E, irradiated, incubated at 10 °C or 30 °C, to model poor refrigeration conditions and severe temperature abuse respectively, and checked daily for off-odours indicative of spoilage and for toxin production. Type E was selected because of its capacity to grow and produce toxin at lower temperatures than other types of *Clostridium botulinum*. It is associated primarily with marine products, but chickens may be fed fish meal containing it (Anon., 1990).

Although toxin was produced in the nonirradiated control chicken, none was found in irradiated chicken held at 10 °C. This difference may be attributable to a reduced ability to produce toxin as a result of radiation damage to the spores. Both irradiated and nonirradiated chicken stored at 30 °C developed toxin. However, chicken irradiated at 3 kGy did not develop toxin under any storage conditions before off-odours characteristic of spoilage became apparent.

In another study (Dezfulian & Bartlett, 1987), the aim was to examine the effect of irradiation (3 kGy) on the growth and toxin production of *Clostridium botulinum* types A and B on chicken skin. These *Clostridium* types are more commonly found on chicken than type E. No toxin was formed from types A and B when chicken was stored at 10 °C, whether irradiated or not. At the abuse temperature of 30 °C, toxin was formed in both irradiated and nonirradiated chicken but toxin formation was delayed in irradiated chicken. No toxin was found before off-odours, signalling spoilage of the food, were produced.

These studies collectively demonstrate that a sufficient number of typical spoilage organisms survive poultry irradiation at 3 kGy to cause clear signs of spoilage before botulinum toxin can develop, thus ensuring that irradiation of poultry at this dose does not pose any additional health hazard from *Clostridium botulinum* (Anon., 1990).

The problems associated with the survival of certain microorganisms after irradiation will depend on the nature of the food and the microbial species with which it is associated. An outbreak of botulism involving fish occurred in the Federal Republic of Germany in 1970 (Bach et al., 1971). The fish had been hot-smoked (not irradiated) but, despite this, several people died as a consequence of toxin produced by type E. This incident prompted development of a research programme at the Federal Research Centre for Nutrition to study the effect of storage temperatures and irradiation on toxin formation in fish inoculated with *Clostridium botulinum* type E (Hussain et al., 1977). With large inocula (10^5 spores per gram), no toxin production was found either in nonirradiated fish or fish irradiated at 1 or 2 kGy when stored at 0 °C. Storage at 5 °C resulted in toxin production in both irradiated and non-irradiated samples, but not until after 6–7 weeks of storage. At this temperature, spoilage — as indicated by off-odour — was noticeable after about 2 weeks in non-irradiated samples, 3 weeks in samples irradiated at 1 kGy, and 4 weeks in samples irradiated at 2 kGy. When fish were stored at 10 °C, however, toxin production occurred before off-odour indicated a hazard.

The large inoculum of 10^5 spores per gram used in these experiments greatly exaggerates any possible hazard. When 10^3 spores per gram were inoculated, no toxin was found in irradiated fish even after 8 weeks of storage at 5 °C, i.e. long after noticeable spoilage. As a matter of prudence, it is recommended that irradiated fish be stored at temperatures of 3 °C or lower to ensure the absence of botulinum toxin in fish throughout its storage life (WHO, 1977).

As both the vegetative form of the organism and its toxin are sensitive to heat, no hazard exists from fish that has been cooked, as would normally be the case for irradiated fish. Smoked fish, on the other hand, is consumed raw, and therefore presents a much greater risk of botulinum poisoning.

In this connection, it should be borne in mind that selective killing and preferential growth of microflora are not unique to irradiation (Department of Health and Human Services, 1984). All nonsterilizing treatments favour the survival and the growth of particular microbial species (Department of Health and Human Services, 1984). For example, *Listeria* and *Yersinia* are capable of growth at low temperatures which suppress the growth of many other organisms (Diehl, 1990), vacuum packing favours the growth of anaerobic species, and salting that of halophilic species.

Although differential growth of pathogens such as *Clostridium botulinum* may result from the irradiation of food, this does not give rise to any special hazards unique to irradiation or any that cannot be effectively managed by means of microbiological and other conventional techniques. In general, the problems encountered with irradiated food appear to be less serious than those found with certain other nonsterilizing processes such as, for example, the smoking of fish (Diehl, 1990).

7.3 Mutations

Concern has been expressed that irradiation will result in the increased induction of mutations in microorganisms (Australian House of Representatives, 1988). Such mutants might be more pathogenic or more virulent, they might be more radiation-resistant, and thus able to survive subsequent food irradiation, or they might pose problems of identification and diagnosis.

It has been known for more than 50 years that ionizing radiation increases the rate of mutation in living organisms (Muller, 1928). While the theoretical possibility that mutation might cause a nonpathogenic organism to be transformed into a pathogenic one or a less virulent strain into a more virulent one cannot be denied, surveys of the scientific literature have uncovered no evidence of such an occurrence. Conversely, it has been shown that irradiation can result in loss of virulence and infectivity (Ingram & Farkas, 1977; Farkas, 1988). This is not surprising, given that the vast majority of mutants are less well adapted to their environment and are less competitive than their wild-type counterparts in the absence of continuing irradiation. Consequently, such mutants would be expected to be at a disadvantage as they attempt to compete in an irradiation-free environment. While mutation, in theory, could lead to unexpected results, including increased pathogenicity, irradiation is by no means unique in being able to increase the rate of mutation. Thermal processing, food preservatives and even drying can all increase mutation rates in microorganisms (Moseley, 1992), yet no evidence has been found to indicate that these forms of food preservation increase the virulence of pathogenic microorganisms. Consequently, there is no scientific basis for the view that irradiation of food will lead to the development of organisms of increased pathogenicity. The only data available on this subject indicate that irradiation would tend to reduce the pathogenicity of foodborne organisms (Ingram & Farkas, 1977).

Another concern (Murray, 1990) is that radiation-resistant mutants might develop, as discussed by Moseley (1992). The use of ionizing irradiation as a food-treatment process might lead to the induction of mutations in contaminating bacteria and to the development of radiation resistance in survivors. In practice, it is extremely difficult to induce such mutations, especially by a single irradiation treatment.

The only successful method for identifying the biochemical pathways for the repair of radiation-induced DNA damage in bacteria has been to isolate mutants that are more resistant to radiation than the wild type or parent strain and then to compare mutants and wild type biochemically. Technically, the isolation of radiation-resistant mutants is easy; if a dose of radiation is applied to a wild-type population so that only a small fraction survives, spontaneous and induced radiation-resistant mutants should be among the survivors. In spite of this, however, very few resistant mutants have been isolated. An exception is the strain *E.coli* B/r isolated from the wild type *E. coli* B (Witkin, 1947). However, this mutant has approximately the same resistance as the wild type K12 strain, *E. coli* AB1157 (Howard-Flanders et al., 1964). This almost total failure to isolate radiation-resistant mutants from a wild type population suggests that wild types of natural strains of bacteria have already evolved an adequate DNA repair capacity. This augurs well for the use of ionizing radiation as a method of pasteurizing food and food ingredients by means of a single radiation treatment.

It is possible to develop radiation-resistant populations by subjecting bacteria to many cycles of irradiation. In these experiments, survivors from a single irradiation treatment are grown to give a large population which is then reirradiated . The survivors from this treatment are again grown and irradiated and so on. After many such rounds of treatment, the population as a whole has, on occasions, been shown to be more resistant than the original one. Genetic analysis of such populations has not generally been carried out. An exception is a radiation-resistant strain of *Salmonella typhimurium* isolated as described above in which mutations were found in two genes as compared with its respective wild type (Ibe et al., 1982). However, in an irradiation plant, food items would necessarily be enclosed in wrapping to prevent recontamination and would be irradiated only once so that the radiation-resistant organisms would not be selected. Radiation is not unique in this respect; heat-resistant mutants of *Salmonella* can be isolated after many cycles of exposure to heat, but ... ms for pasteurizing plants which have been operating for almost 100 years.

Another possibility is that radiation might change the properties of pathogenic organisms so dramatically that they might escape proper identification. It is clear, however, that the vast majority of the characteristics of microorganisms remain unchanged after mutation has occurred, making their identification by the usual methods easily possible (Finegold & Martin, 1982). Ingram & Farkas (1977), who closely examined this issue, found nothing to suggest that a problem exists. It is particularly reassuring that radiation has been used extensively in medicine for many years, both for diagnostic and therapeutic purposes and for sterilizing equipment and medical devices, yet no evidence of diagnostic problems attributable to its use has emerged.

7.4 Mycotoxin production

Jemmali & Guilbot (1969), Applegate & Chipley (1973) and Priyadarshini & Tulpule (1979) reported an increase in the production of aflatoxin by *Aspergillus flavus* and *Aspergillus parasiticus* following irradiation of their spores. Paster et al. (1985) reported an increase in ochratoxin after irradiation of *Aspergillus ochraceus*. Other investigators (Ingram & Farkas, 1977) have found that irradiation decreased rather than increased aflatoxin production. The variability of these results may be a consequence of the very nature of *Aspergillus*, which is heterokaryotic, so that different nuclei within a mycelium can undergo exchange with the mycelium of a different strain and thereby acquire new characteristics. This enables subcultures to have different properties, such as higher or lower aflatoxin-producing ability, in comparison with the parent strain. Also confounding the results is the dependence of toxin formation on the size of the inoculum which, according to Diehl (1990), was not taken into account in many of the studies reported.

Sharma et al. (1980) and Odamtten et al. (1987) conclusively demonstrated the role played by inoculum size in aflatoxin production. A reduction by a factor of 10^4 in the number of spores, whether caused by simple dilution or radiation, resulted in a two-fold increase in aflatoxin production by *Aspergillus parasiticus* and up to a 12-fold increase in such production by *Aspergillus flavus*.

In a field trial by Behere et al. (1978), naturally contaminated wheat was stored under conditions of 90% relative humidity at 28 °C. Lower levels of aflatoxin were found in irradiated samples than in nonirradiated controls. Frank et al. (1971) studied the effects of repeated cycles of sublethal irradiation on the growth of *Aspergillus flavus*, and found that irradiation more frequently led to a complete loss or decrease of aflatoxin production than to an increase.

irradiated and stored under ... data indicate that food ... be at no increased risk of producing aflatoxin.

7.5 Summary and conclusions

The existing body of scientific evidence indicates that irradiation produces no problems that have not already been recognized and addressed for other forms of food processing designed to reduce the number of microbes or to destroy pathogenic organisms. Consideration of the microbiological safety of irradiated food, therefore, raises the same issues that arise with all accepted nonsterilizing methods of food processing and are amenable to the same standard techniques as those used to determine microbiologically safe conditions for traditional types of food processing. There is no reason, therefore, for food, once irradiated at nonsterilizing doses, to be subjected to any controls other than those typically applied to food treated by traditional nonsterilizing processes used either to extend shelf-life or to destroy pathogens.

At the request of the WHO Secretary of the Codex Alimentarius Commission, the issue of the microbiological safety of irradiated food was again reviewed in December 1982 by a group of internationally renowned food microbiologists belonging to the International Committee on Food Microbiology and Hygiene. The conclusion of this group was that food irradiation should be seen as an important addition to existing methods of control of foodborne pathogens and did not present any additional hazards to health (FAO, 1983).

References

Advisory Committee on Irradiated and Novel Foods (1986) *Report on the safety and wholesomeness of irradiated foods.* London, Her Majesty's Stationery Office.

Anon. (1990) Irradiation in the production, processing and handling of food. Final rule. *Federal register,* **55**: 18544

Anon. (1991) Irradiation in the production, processing and handling of food. In: *Code of federal regulations.* Title 21, Part 179.

Applegate KL, Chipley JR (1973) Increased aflatoxin G_1 production by *Aspergillus flavus* via gamma irradiation. *Mycologia,* **65**: 1266–1273.

Australian House of Representatives (Standing Committee on Environment, Recreation and the Arts) (1988) *Use of ionising radiation.* Canberra, Australian Government Publishing Service.

Bach R et al. (1971) [Trout from ponds as a carrier of *Clostridium botulinum* and cause of botulism. Part 3.] *Archiv für Lebensmittelhygiene*, 22:107–112 (in German).

Behere AG et al. (1978) Production of aflatoxins during storage of gamma-irradiated wheat. *Journal of food science*, 43:1102–1103.

Department of Health and Human Services (1984) *Proceedings of the Second National Conference for Food Protection*. Washington, DC, pp. 103–217.

Dezfulian M, Bartlett JG (1987) Effect of irradiation on growth and toxigenicity of *Clostridium botulinum* types A and B inoculated onto chicken skins. *Applied and environmental microbiology*, 53:201–203.

Diehl JF (1990) *Safety of irradiated food*. New York, Marcel Dekker, pp. 181–193.

FAO (1983) *The microbiological safety of irradiated food*. Rome, Food and Agriculture Organization of the United Nations (unpublished document of the Codex Alimentarius Commission, No. CX/FH 83/9).

Farkas J (1988) *Irradiation of dry food ingredients*. Boca Raton, FL, CRC Press, p. 57.

Finegold SM, Martin WJ (1982) *Diagnostic microbiology*, 6th ed. St Louis, Toronto, London, CV Mosby.

Firstenberg-Eden R et al. (1983) Competitive growth of chicken skin microflora and *Clostridium botulinum* type E after an irradiation dose of 0.3 Mrad. *Journal of food protection*, 46:12–15.

Frank HK et al. (1971) Response of toxigenic and non-toxigenic strains of *Aspergillus flavus* to irradiation. *Sabouraudia*, 9:21–26.

Howard-Flanders P et al. (1964) A locus that controls filament formation and sensitivity to irradiation in *Escherichia coli* K-12. *Genetics*, 49: 237.

Hussain AM et al. (1977) Comparison of toxin production by *Clostridium botulinum* type E in irradiated and unirradiated vacuum-packed trout (*Salmo gairdneri*). *Archiv für Lebensmittelhygiene*, 28:23–27.

Ibe SN et al. (1982) Genetic mapping of mutations in a highly radiation-resistant mutant of *Salmonella typhimurium* LT2. *Journal of bacteriology*, 152:260.

Ingram M, Farkas J (1977) Microbiology of foods pasteurised by ionising radiation. *Acta alimentaria*, 6:123–185.

Jemmali M, Guilbot A (1969) Influence de l'irradiation des spores d'*A. flavus* sur la production d'aflatoxin B. *Comptes rendus hebdomadaires des seances de l'Academie des Sciences (Paris)*, **269** Ser. D: 2271–2273.

Käferstein FK (1990) Food irradiation and its role in improving the safety and security of food. *Food control*, **1**(4): 211–214.

Licciardello JJ et al. (1968) Elimination of *Salmonella* in poultry with ionizing radiation. In: *Elimination of harmful organisms from food and feed by irradiation*. Vienna, International Atomic Energy Agency (Panel Proceedings Series), pp. 1–28.

Matches JR, Liston J (1971) Radiation destruction of *Vibrio parahaemolyticus*. *Journal of food science*, **36**: 339–340.

Maxcy RG (1983) Significance of residual organisms in foods after substerilizing doses of gamma radiation: a review. *Journal of food safety*, **5**: 203–211.

Maxcy RB & Tiwari NP (1973) Irradiation of meats for public health protection. In: *Radiation preservation of food. Proceedings of a Symposium held in Bombay, November 1972*. Vienna, International Atomic Energy Agency, pp. 491–503.

Moseley B (1992) Radiation, microorganisms and radiation resistance. In: Johnston DE, Stevenson MH, eds. *Food irradiation and the chemist*. Cambridge, Royal Society of Chemistry, pp. 97–108 (Publication No. 86).

Mossel DAA, Stegeman H (1985) Irradiation: an effective mode of processing food for safety. In: *Food irradiation processing. Proceedings of a Symposium held in Washington, DC, March 1985*. Vienna, International Atomic Energy Agency, p. 251.

Mulder RWAW (1982) *Radicidation of poultry carcasses*. Beekbergen, The Netherlands, Spelderholt Institute for Poultry Research (Report No. 363).

Muller HJ (1928) Mutations induced in *Drosophila*. *Genetics*, **13**: 279.

Murray DR (1990) *Biology of food irradiation*. New York, John Wiley.

Odamtten GT et al. (1987) Influence of inoculum size of *Aspergillus flavus* Link on the production of B_1 in maize medium before and after exposure to combination treatment of heat and gamma radiation. *International journal of food microbiology*, **4**: 119–127.

Palumbo SA et al. (1986) Determination of irradiation D-values for *Aeromonas hydrophila*. *Journal of food protection*, **49**: 189–191.

Paster N et al. (1985) Effect of gamma radiation on ochratoxin production by the fungus *Aspergillus ochraceus. Journal of the science of food and agriculture*, **36**: 445–449.

Priyadarshini E, Tulpule PG (1979) Effect of graded doses of gamma-irradiation on aflatoxin production by *Aspergillus parasiticus* in wheat. *Food and cosmetic toxicology*, **17**, 505–507.

Quinn DJ et al. (1967) The inactivation of infection and intoxication microorganisms by irradiation in seafood. In: *Microbiological problems in food preservation by irradiation.* Vienna, International Atomic Energy Agency, p. 1 (Panel Proceedings Series).

Rowley DB et al. (1983) Radiation-injured *Clostridium botulinum* type E spores: outgrowth and repair. *Journal of food science*, **48**: 1829–1831.

Sharma A et al. (1980) Influence of inoculum size of *Aspergillus parasiticus* spores on aflatoxin production. *Applied and environmental microbiology*, **40**: 989–993.

Tarkowski JA et al. (1984) Low dose gamma irradiation of raw meat. I. Bacteriological and sensory quality effects in artificially contaminated samples. *International journal of food microbiology*, **1**: 13–23.

WHO (1977) *Wholesomeness of irradiated food. Report of a Joint FAO/IAEA/WHO Expert Committee*. Geneva, World Health Organization (WHO Technical Report Series, No. 604).

Witkin EM (1947) Genetics of resistance to radiation in *Escherichia coli. Genetics*, **32**: 221.

8.
Nutritional quality

8.1 Introduction

This chapter examines what is known about the nutritional quality of irradiated foods, including possible research needs and key references from which conclusions as to nutritional quality can be drawn. For practical purposes, the discussion concentrates on the nutritional evaluation of foods treated with low (up to 1 kGy) and medium (1–10 kGy) radiation doses. The effects of high-dose irradiation are mentioned where this helps to clarify specific points. As discussed in detail in Chapter 3, low-dose irradiation is primarily aimed at inhibition of sprouting, delaying of the maturation of fresh produce, the destruction or sexual sterilization of insects, and the destruction of parasites. Medium-dose irradiation is aimed primarily at reducing or eliminating bacteria, yeasts and moulds that can act as human pathogens or hasten spoilage or both. This differentiation between dose levels is well described elsewhere (WHO, 1988).

As far as high-dose irradiation (approximately 10–45 kGy) is concerned, the United States Army has historically been the principal contributor to research and development, because of its interest in readily available meat, poultry, fish and shellfish of good nutritional quality that can withstand prolonged storage at ambient temperatures. Food subjected to such high-dose irradiation can also be used to increase the variety of items available to immunocompromised patients requiring sterile environments, and the process has been employed to a limited extent to produce food for critically ill patients for several decades. During the 1980s, however, the United States Army ceased to take a major interest in irradiation-sterilized food products, largely because its needs were met, e.g. by flex-packaged, thermally processed products; these are of good quality and have some logistic advantages. However, in 1992, the United States Army was reconsidering possible further study of irradiation-sterilized foods for special uses. Few other groups have shown a sustained interest in irradiation sterilization, and the practical value of this type of food processing from the point of view of the general population is doubtful for the foreseeable future. However, it is worthy of note that, even with such high-dose processing, nutrient losses are generally not of major significance if processing is properly carried out, e.g. by irradiation in the frozen state coupled with appropriate packaging.

8. NUTRITIONAL QUALITY

8.2 Synopsis of reviews

8.2.1 International reviews

A meeting of a Joint FAO/IAEA/WHO Expert Committee on the Wholesomeness of Irradiated Food (WHO, 1981) was particularly important from a nutritional point of view because the Committee concluded that "irradiation of food up to an overall average dose of 10 kGy introduces no special nutritional or microbiological problems."

8.2.2 National and regional reviews

United Kingdom

In 1986, the Advisory Committee on Irradiated and Novel Foods, a joint committee established by the Department of Health and Social Security and the Ministry of Agriculture, Fisheries and Food, issued a report entitled *Report on the safety and wholesomeness of irradiated foods*, in which the following three statements are particularly worthy of note (Advisory Committee on Irradiated and Novel Foods, 1986):

> The studies showed a reduction in the content of some vitamins in many irradiated food classes comparable to the reductions caused by other methods of processing food.
> The nutritional consequences of food irradiation are not qualitatively or quantitatively different from the nutritional consequences of currently accepted methods of processing and preparing foods.
> We consider that the irradiation of food up to an overall average dose of 10 kGy introduces no special nutritional problems.

Canada, Denmark and Sweden

All three countries have issued reports on the wholesomeness of irradiated foods (Health and Welfare Canada, 1987; Ministry of Agriculture, 1983; National Food Agency, 1986), which generally support the conclusions reached at the meeting of the Joint FAO/IAEA/WHO Expert Committee in 1980.

United States of America

The results, reviews and reports of nutrition research, and Congressional testimonies regarding the nutritional quality of irradiated foods, are primarily housed in the archives of the United States Army Natick Laboratories, Natick, MA, and the FDA. The latter established an Irradiated Foods Committee in 1979 and its successor, the Irradiated Foods Task Force, in 1981, primarily to develop regulatory responses to petitions being received for low-dose and medium-dose applications, many of which have now been approved.

Commission of the European Communities

In 1987, the Scientific Committee on Food (1987) of the Commission of the European Communities gave advice to the Commission in support of the conclusions reached at the meeting of the Joint FAO/IAEA/WHO Expert Committee in 1980, including those concerning the nutritional aspects, and reaffirmed that no further animal feeding studies were needed to assess the safety of food irradiated up to a dose of 10 kGy.

It is important to keep in mind that, in considering the "wholesomeness" of food, nutritional quality is just as much a component as are toxicological parameters, the absence of contamination, and the like. This concept forms the core of all of the various reviews on irradiated foods, whether by the specialized agencies of the United Nations, government bodies or the scientific community.

8.2.3 Reviews by the scientific community

A number of reviews of food irradiation have been published over the past 10 years or so. *Preservation of food by ionizing irradiation* (Josephson & Peterson, 1982), deals primarily with high-dose irradiation for sterilization purposes. It contains the following passage:

> From the foregoing discussion, we have seen that irradiation at sterilizing and near-sterilizing doses does degrade a variety of nutrients. However, the overall effect is not significant since radiation is not unique in this respect, and various studies have shown that the sterilization of foods with thermal energy has equally destructive effects on their nutrient components. To put it another way, the use of radiation for preserving foods does not degrade their nutritional quality more than it is degraded by preserving them with heat.

A paper published in 1983, entitled "Nutritional aspects of food irradiation" (Murray, 1983), contained the following statement: "None of the evidence reviewed necessitates a change in the advice on the nutritional aspects of food irradiation given by the 1976 Joint FAO/IAEA/WHO Expert Committee."

The publication *Safety of irradiated foods* (Diehl, 1990) is concerned primarily with low-dose and medium-dose irradiation. Chapter 7 of this book, entitled "Nutritional adequacy of irradiated foods", contains the following statement: "As with regard to potential microbiological problems . . . it can be stated that potential nutritional losses in irradiated foods are not basically different from losses in foods treated by other processes. On the contrary, heating, drying, and some other traditional methods may cause higher nutritional losses than irradiation."

In addition, Professor Diehl and his colleagues have recently published two reviews devoted entirely to nutritional aspects, entitled respectively "Nutritional effects of combining irradiation with other treatments" (Diehl,

1991) and "Regulation of food irradiation in the European Community: is nutrition an issue?" (Diehl et al., 1991). The former provides data to substantiate the conclusion that losses of radiation-sensitive vitamins can be minimized either by oxygen-free packaging at the time of irradiation or by irradiation at cryogenic temperatures, or both. The latter provides recent data on all macronutrients, which are not significantly affected, and on vitamins, several of which may suffer losses to varying degrees. The paper concludes that "The loss is no greater and is usually smaller than that following accepted processing methods, such as canning."

8.2.4 Conclusions

Individual research and reviews at all levels have led to the conclusion that low-dose and medium-dose irradiation of conventional foods results in foods of good nutritional quality which are wholesome in all respects. Such foods are equivalent to foods processed by other means such as drying, smoking, canning and freezing. Losses of radiation-sensitive vitamins can be minimized by means of appropriate processing techniques.

8.3 Nutrient levels

In view of the complex matrix of variables involved, it is small wonder that investigations of the effects of ionizing radiation on nutritional quality are sometimes difficult to interpret. Few of the many hundreds of studies carried out have covered the same set of variables, and some of the variables have often been outside the realm of the practical application of irradiation, e.g. very high radiation doses. This matrix of variables includes:

— purpose of the study;
— radiation dose;
— radiation source;
— temperature;
— hydration;
— individual nutrients;
— atmosphere at the time of irradiation;
— storage conditions;
— antimetabolites; and
— the food itself.

These are discussed further below.

8.3.1 Purpose of study

A large proportion of the studies that have examined nutritional quality were undertaken primarily for other reasons, usually to assess the impact on overall quality of irradiating to achieve specific goals, such as the prolongation of shelf-life, disinfestation, and sterilization. This alone tends to fragment the literature concerned with nutrition.

8.3.2 Radiation dose

The dose of radiation necessary to achieve the intended purpose varies over a very wide range, from 0.1 kGy to 60 kGy or even higher. In all the ranges — low-dose, medium-dose, and high-dose—there is a lack of consistency in the doses actually applied from study to study. This inconsistency simply has to be accepted in interpreting the impact on nutrient levels. A common error has been to assume that the effects on nutrient levels at one dose are applicable at other levels.

8.3.3 Radiation source

Fortunately, not many examples of differences in nutrient levels depend on the radiation source, but there are a few. For example, in pork irradiated at 60 kGy and $-45°C$, thiamine is much better preserved with electron irradiation than with gamma sources (Thomas et al., 1981). This is thought to be due to the fact that a much higher dose rate (at the same total dose) is delivered by the electron beam. At low-dose and medium-dose levels, there is no evidence that significant differences exist between the radiation sources.

8.3.4 Temperature

Heat

Diehl reports that a combination of dipping in hot water and irradiation considerably improves the shelf-life of some fruits without adversely affecting vitamin C levels (Diehl, 1981).

Many foods are cooked after irradiation, as happens with foods preserved by other techniques. The combined effects of irradiation and cooking must be considered in order to assess accurately the quality of the food when it is actually consumed. There is a paucity of data on the nutrient content of cooked irradiated foods, but this is also true for a great many foods processed in other ways. For this reason, most nutrition labelling indicates the nutrient content at the time of purchase. A major reason for this lack of data is the simple fact that the enormous variations in cooking practices make it virtually impossible to document accurately the extent of nutrient losses in a meaningful manner. Those few studies that are available on irradiated foods suggest that cooking, e.g. boiling, steaming, or baking, has a greater negative impact on vitamin levels than low-dose or medium-dose irradiation, as illustrated in Table 15 (Sreenivasan, 1974).

Table 15. Effect of radiation and cooking on retention of B vitamins in red gram (Cajanus cajan), a major staple food in south Asia

Treatment	Retention (%)		
	Riboflavin	Thiamine	Niacin
Irradiated (10 kGy, uncooked)	98.7	92.7	93.3
Control (cooked)	88.0	76.1	83.3
Irradiated (10 kGy, cooked)	95.0	82.7	89.3

Source: Adapted from Sreenivasan (1974).

Cold

Early in the studies by the United States Army of irradiation-sterilized (high-dose) meat, poultry and seafood, it was learned that the use of cryogenic temperatures during irradiation had a major beneficial effect on the retention of many vitamins. This also applied to low-dose and medium-dose irradiation, as illustrated in Table 16.

Generally speaking, most research indicates that temperatures in the range $-20\,°C$ to $-40\,°C$ are sufficient to minimize vitamin losses.

8.3.5 Hydration

Aqueous and other solutions of some vitamins are highly vulnerable to destruction by irradiation, but this is not true of vitamins in foods themselves. Generally speaking, the irradiation of dehydrated foods leads to substantially less nutrient loss than that of foods containing their normal amount of water. As an example, thiamine in aqueous solution (2.5 mg/l) suffered a 50% loss

Table 16. Effect of temperature during irradiation on retention of α-tocopherol in rolled oats[a]

Temperature (°C)	α-Tocopherol (mg/100 g)		Decrease (%)
	Nonirradiated	Irradiated	
50	6.5	3.5	46
20	7.4	5.6	24
5	7.5	6.2	17
−72	7.7	6.6	14
−180	7.6	7.1	7

[a]Linear accelerator, 5 MeV electrons, 1 kGy, air not excluded; analysis within 24 hours after irradiation.
Source: Diehl (1981)

after irradiation with a dose of 0.5 kGy, while irradiation of dried whole egg containing 3.9 mg of thiamine per kg with the same dose caused less than 5% destruction (Diehl, 1975). It is inappropriate to extrapolate data on nutrient loss from individual vitamins in solution to food.

An interesting aspect of the effects of irradiating dried food is that the subsequent cooking time of the rehydrated, irradiated legumes is reduced, resulting in improved vitamin retention (Sreenivasan, 1974). Another general observation is that loss of vitamin C from irradiated dried vegetable products is minimal. In fact, no loss at all was observed in onion powder even when the extremely high dose of 270 kGy was used for samples in tin cans, and a dose of 20 kGy for samples irradiated in commercial boxes (Galetto et al., 1979). As pointed out by Murray (1983), the vitamins in spices are generally very resistant to irradiation, e.g. irradiation of paprika at 0–22 °C with doses of 5–50 kGy and subsequent storage for 6 months had practically no effect on the levels of carotenoids. This, in itself, is not nutritionally significant since spices do not make a major nutrient contribution to the total diet. Irradiated spices are now commercially available in a number of countries.

8.3.6 Individual nutrients

Macronutrients

At the low and medium doses under consideration here, there are no significant effects on the nutritional value of proteins, carbohydrates, or fats (Diehl, 1990, 1991; Diehl et al., 1991). This is usually also true with higher doses, depending on the specific food being irradiated and the environmental conditions. These conclusions have been well established *in vivo* by numerous animal studies, including measurements of the protein efficiency ratio (PER) for many irradiated foods providing significant amounts of protein, including those irradiated at sterilizing doses. This is the fundamental reason why it has been so difficult to find a chemicoanalytical indicator that would make it possible to determine whether a food has or has not been irradiated (see Chapter 5).

The question of possible destruction of polyunsaturated fatty acids has been studied by a number of investigators. When whole-grain cereals (wheat, rice and rye) were irradiated at 0.1–1 kGy, no losses of unsaturated fatty acids were observed (Vaca & Harms-Ringdahl, 1986). Only small losses were found even at the very high dose of 63 kGy. The irradiation of herring fillets at sterilizing doses (50 kGy) also had no effect on the content of polyunsaturated fatty acids (Adam et al., 1982). Some destruction was observed when a mixture of herring oil and starch was irradiated and stored in air (Hammer & Wills, 1979). However, there is no food that would correspond to this artificial mixture, and the observation is therefore of doubtful practical significance.

Essential minerals

There is no evidence that irradiation, regardless of dose, has any effect on essential minerals, in terms of either amount or bioavailability.

Water-soluble vitamins

There is a very large body of scientific literature on the effects of irradiation on the retention and destruction of the water-soluble vitamins (Josephson & Peterson, 1982; Murray, 1983; Diehl, 1990; Diehl et al., 1991). Although effects on vitamin levels vary from food to food, the order of sensitivity to irradiation is generally as follows: thiamine > ascorbic acid > pyridoxine > riboflavin > folic acid > cobalamin > nicotinic acid. In the interpretation of individual research results, it is also important to keep in mind that natural variation in vitamin content is substantial, depending on many factors, such as plant and animal variety, season of the year and storage conditions.

Until recently, there has been a paucity of good data on the effects of irradiation on folic acid. However, Muller (1991) has recently presented data indicating some loss of tetrahydrofolic acid in pulses after irradiation at the high dose of 25 kGy, but no effect on levels of folic acid, dihydrofolic acid, 5-methyltetrahydrofolic acid, and 4-formyltetrahydrofolic acid. These results need to be independently confirmed, and the studies extended to other classes of foods.

Diehl et al. (1991) have recently summarized the results of studies on cobalamin indicating that this vitamin is relatively resistant to irradiation. Data were reviewed both for animal-derived foods (haddock fillets at 25 kGy, pork chops at up to 6.65 kGy), and for dairy products (40 kGy in a nitrogen atmosphere). No losses of cyanocobalamin were observed in any of these studies over a wide range of dose.

Data on the effect of irradiation on some of the major B vitamins in cod, packed in polyethylene bags without exclusion of air, are given in Table 17 (Kennedy & Ley, 1971). These results show the relatively high radiation-sensitivity of thiamine as compared with nicotinic acid and riboflavin. As mentioned in sections 8.3.7 and 8.3.8, losses of thiamine can be greatly reduced by exclusion of air during irradiation and storage. For further details, the reader is referred particularly to the reviews by Murray (1983) and Diehl et al. (1991).

With regard to vitamin C, it is important to remember that many of the earlier studies on losses of this vitamin used relatively high doses of radiation and measured only ascorbic acid itself, with the result that major decreases in vitamin C activity were reported. As emphasized by Diehl (1990) and by Diehl et al. (1991), total vitamin C activity is the sum of the activities of ascorbic acid and dehydroascorbic acid. It is quite true that irradiation may result in increased amounts of dehydroascorbic acid with concomitant decreases in ascorbic acid, but this is of no nutritional significance since both

Table 17. Effect of irradiation (at 6 kGy) and cooking (4 min at 100 kPa) on some B-complex vitamins in cod[a]

Treatment	Retention (%)		
	Nicotinic acid	Riboflavin	Thiamine
Raw cod	100	100	100
Irradiated raw	99	94	53
Non-irradiated, cooked	96	91	90
Irradiated, cooked	97	84	46

[a]Adapted from a table by Diehl (1990) based on Kennedy & Ley (1971).

substances are of equal biological activity. Typical examples of the effects on vitamin C are: (1) those reported by Fesus et al. (1981), who found that oranges treated with 0.4, 0.6 or 0.8 kGy had approximately the same concentration of vitamin C 1 or 2 days after treatment; and (2) those reported by Nagay & Moy (1985) for oranges irradiated with 0.3, 0.5, 0.75 and 1.0 kGy and stored for 7 weeks at 7 °C, which also did not differ significantly from nonirradiated fruits in vitamin C content. When consideration is being given to marketing irradiated foods that make major contributions to vitamin C intake, it is important also to measure the vitamin content in the irradiated product under the storage conditions expected.

Fat-soluble vitamins

As with the water-soluble vitamins, the sensitivity to radiation of the fat-soluble vitamins varies greatly depending on the specific food involved, the radiation dose, and the environmental conditions during irradiation and storage. Nevertheless, it can be stated that, in general, the order of sensitivity is as follows: vitamin E > carotene > vitamin A > vitamin K > vitamin D.

The radiation-sensitivity of vitamin E depends greatly on the presence of oxygen during irradiation and storage. When rolled oats were irradiated with a dose of 1 kGy and stored in the presence of air, they had 44% less vitamin E than the unirradiated control samples after 6 months of storage. Packaging under nitrogen reduced the loss to 7% (Diehl, 1979b). The main sources of vitamin E in the human diet are butter, margarine and fats and oils of plant origin. None of these foods is suitable for commercial irradiation.

When pork liver was treated with 5 kGy at 0 °C and stored at the same temperature, it contained 4% less vitamin A than the non-irradiated control after one week, and 13% less after four weeks. Calf liver sausage showed losses of 10% and 18% respectively under the same conditions. Powdered whole egg irradiated with 10 kGy lost 22% of its vitamin A in four weeks when packaged in air, and 6% in vacuum (Diehl, 1979a). Vitamin A was unaffected in dogfish fillets irradiated at 0 °C with 3 kGy; 45% was lost after treatment with 30 kGy (Mameesh et al., 1964). Most of the foods that are important sources of vitamin A in the human diet, such as milk, butter and cheese, are unlikely candidates for commercial food irradiation.

While preformed vitamin A is found only in foods of animal origin, β-carotene and some other carotenoids found in vegetables and fruits can be converted to vitamin A in the human body. The effect of irradiation on the carotenoids has been studied extensively, and the results differ considerably in different products. No effect was seen on the concentration of β-carotene in mandarins and pineapple on irradiation with 2.45 kGy (Agneessens et al., 1989). Freshly milled flour from wheat irradiated with 1 kGy showed 2–7% lower carotenoid concentrations than flour from non-irradiated wheat (Tipples & Norris, 1965). In potatoes irradiated with 0.1 kGy, no loss of carotenoids was seen immediately after irradiation. During six months of storage, the carotenoids decreased to about 50% of their initial value, whereas no change or an increase was seen in non-irradiated potatoes (Janave & Thomas, 1979).

For further details and for data on the more radiation-stable vitamins D and K, see the reviews by Murray (1983) and Diehl et al. (1991).

8.3.7 Atmosphere at the time of irradiation

As discussed earlier, a higher proportion of the vitamin content is preserved if food is irradiated at low temperature. The same is true if irradiation takes place in an oxygen-free environment, something that is particularly applicable to vitamins that are radiation-sensitive, such as thiamine, ascorbic acid and α-tocopherol. In practice, this involves irradiating under vacuum or using nitrogen flushing during irradiation and packaging. Even when high radiation doses are used, vitamin losses can be kept to a minimum by choosing appropriate conditions, as shown in Table 18.

8.3.8 Storage conditions

Storage conditions are important for irradiated foods, as they are for all other forms of preserved food. Even thermally processed foods in cans must be stored under reasonable conditions to preserve their nutrient content over extended periods. For example, prolonged storage of canned infant formulas (as well as dry packed formulas) in extremely hot environments has resulted in dangerous nutrient deterioration. Many irradiated foods, especially when irradiated at low doses, are stable under ordinary conditions without any special handling, but other irradiated foods, e.g. fresh fruits, require refrigeration, as do their nonirradiated counterparts, to preserve both their organoleptic properties and nutrient content.

Table 18. Vitamin contents of frozen, thermally processed, gamma-irradiated, and electron-irradiated enzyme-inactivated chicken meat[a]

Vitamin	Vitamin concentration, dry weight (mg/kg)[b]			
	Frozen control	Heat-sterilized	Gamma-irradiated[c]	Electron irradiated[c]
Thiamine-HCl	2.31	1.53[d]	1.57[d]	1.98
Riboflavin	4.32	4.60	4.46	4.90[e]
Pyridoxine	7.26	7.62	5.32	6.70
Nicotinic acid	212.9	213.9	197.9	208.2
Panothenic acid	24.0	21.8	23.5	24.9
Biotin	0.093	0.097	0.098	0.103
Folic acid	0.83	1.22	1.26	1.47[e]
Vitamin A	2716	2340	2270	2270
Vitamin D	375.1	342.8	354.0	466.1
Vitamin K	1.29	1.01	0.81	0.85
Vitamin B_{12}	0.008	0.016[e]	0.014[e]	0.009

[a]Adapted from Thayer (1990).
[b]Concentrations of vitamin D and vitamin K are given as IU/kg.
[c]58 kGy at 25°C
[d]Significantly lower than frozen control.
[e]Significantly higher than frozen control.

As an example of the effect of storage conditions, rolled oats irradiated at 0.25 kGy lost about one-quarter of their thiamine content after 4 months of storage in air, but virtually none if stored in nitrogen (Diehl, 1981). The same was true for vitamin E in rolled oats irradiated at 1 kGy and stored for 8 months (Diehl, 1990). Murray (1983) reached the following conclusion regarding endives irradiated at a dose of 1 kGy: "The best results with regard to keeping quality and vitamin C content were achieved following storage in unperforated polythene bags." Murray also noted that the vitamin content of mackerel, irradiated at 1–45 kGy, was best preserved if it was stored at −22 °C in plastic bags. These examples are further evidence of the complexity of the set of variables involved. Each food under consideration for entry into the general food supply must be evaluated individually and with a clear understanding of all the variables involved, including the conditions of storage throughout the shelf-life of the product and in the home.

8.3.9 Antimetabolites

In the 1970s, concerns arose over the possibility that irradiation-induced antimetabolites might be formed, particularly to thiamine and pyridoxine.

A number of groups investigated this question in experimental animal studies, and no such antimetabolites were found (Murray, 1983; Diehl, 1990). There is no evidence to suggest that antimetabolites are produced in irradiated foods. When vitamin losses occur, it is reasonable to conclude that these are partial losses of the same type as those found with all forms of food preservation.

8.4 Role of irradiated food in the total daily diet

The nutritional significance of vitamin losses induced by irradiation will depend very much on the proportion of irradiated foods in the diet. As long as such foods constitute only a small fraction of the daily food consumption, concern is unwarranted, especially when irradiation is limited to items such as spices, which do not contribute significantly to the vitamin supply. A high proportion of irradiated foods in the daily diet would raise concerns similar to those associated with a high proportion of foods processed in other ways.

Given the complexity of food technology and the decentralization of the production, transport and storage of food commodities, the introduction of irradiated foods into the food supply is likely to be gradual and to extend over a long period, providing ample time for evaluation.

8.5 Preregistration requirements

The preregistration requirements imposed by national or regional food authorities should require the submission of the following data:

1. Nutrient analytical data covering the shelf-life of the product under recommended storage conditions for all vitamins present in nutritionally significant amounts in the food prior to processing. "Significant amounts" are often defined as 5% or more of the recommended daily intakes (RDIs) per serving or portion. As mentioned earlier, there are no indications that macronutrient or mineral contents are altered by irradiation so as to adversely affect the nutritional quality of the food.
2. A description of the anticipated role that the food will play in the total daily diet, in particular in population groups that could reasonably be expected to consume larger amounts than the general population, e.g. toddlers or the elderly.

8.6 Labelling

Labelling is an effective way of providing consumers with information on the maintenance of the quality and safety of food. It is very important when new technologies such as irradiation are being introduced. Such labelling should meet the recommendations specified by the Codex General Standard for the Labelling of Prepackaged Foods (FAO, 1991).

8.7 Postm...

Because irr... ...untries, measurement of... ...ne a part of all food consu... ...such foods in national or... ...ies of this kind are of majo... ...these measurements, nutrition and health authorities do not know what the public is consuming; and (b) considerable errors are often made when reliance is placed on food commodity disappearance data to estimate human consumption, usually on the side of gross overestimates of actual intake.

The requirements suggested in sections 8.5–8.7 are not particular to food irradiation. They should apply to all new food processing technologies and to all novel foods.

8.8 Research needs

There is general agreement that there is no need for further studies on the toxicological aspects of foods irradiated at doses up to 10 kGy. Much the same can be said about nutritional quality at these doses. From a practical point of view, the remaining research needs as far as nutritional factors are concerned are of an applied nature, and can in large measure be met through the supportive measures described above, i.e. preregistration requirements, labelling, and postmarketing surveillance. In this way, a substantial body of data on nutrient composition, of great practical significance, will eventually be generated, reflecting the nutrient composition of foods processed under specified conditions and actually on the market. A fundamental problem with nutrient composition data is that the number of variables to be considered is enormous. Also, as pointed out by Diehl et al. (1991) and Diehl (1991), particular attention should be paid to the study of levels of radiation-sensitive vitamins (particularly thiamine and α-tocopherol) under the processing conditions likely to exist when the foods are marketed.

Basic research to elucidate the mechanisms of the empirically observed nutritional phenomena at doses above 10 kGy, particularly in oxygen-free environments and at cryogenic temperatures, would provide useful information for possible future applications of higher radiation doses.

8.9 Summary and conclusions

Forty years of research have demonstrated that foods can be preserved by ionizing radiation up to a dose of 10 kGy with good nutritional quality. Many reviews of studies on food irradiation have been undertaken at international, national and regional levels and all have reached the same conclusions.

Examination of the nutrient losses that do occur demonstrates that only a few vitamins are adversely affected, particularly thiamine and the tocopherols. At the irradiation conditions recommended, these losses are small, of the order of 10–20% or less, and comparable to those seen with other forms of food preservation, such as thermal processing and drying. Macronutrients and essential minerals are not affected.

In a number of countries, governments have taken a stand in approving the introduction of irradiated food items into the national food supplies. This will be a gradual process, so that there will be ample opportunity to evaluate it from the public health, economic, and consumer points of view.

Maintenance of the nutritional quality of irradiated foods can be facilitated by means of several supportive measures such as preregistration requirements, appropriate labelling, postmarketing surveillance and provision of information on the nutritional quality of specific irradiated foods.

References

Adam S et al. (1982) Influence of ionizing radiation on the fatty acid composition of herring fillets. *Radiation physics and chemistry*, **20**:289–295.

Advisory Committee on Irradiated and Novel Foods (1986) *Report on the safety and wholesomeness of irradiated foods.* London, Her Majesty's Stationery Office.

Agneessens R et al. (1989) Dosage du β-carotène dans les fruits irradiés, par chromatographie liquide à haute performance avec détection ampérométrique. *Bulletin des recherches agronomiques de Gembloux*, **24**: 85–90.

Bierman EL et al. (1958) *Short-term human feeding studies of foods sterilized by gamma radiation and stored at room temperature.* US Army Medical Research and Nutrition Laboratory, Report No. 224, 1 July 1958 (unpublished document; obtainable in microfiche form from Defense Technical Information Center, DTIC-2DA, Cameron Station, Alexandria, VA 22304–6145, USA).

Diehl JF (1975) [Thiamine in irradiated foods. 1. Influence of various conditions and of time after irradiation.] *Zeitschrift für Lebensmittel-Untersuchung und -Forschung*, **157**:317–321 (in German).

Diehl JF (1979a) Vitamin A in bestrahlten Lebensmitteln. *Zeitschrift für Lebensmittel-Untersuchung und -Forschung*, **168**:29–31.

Diehl JF (1979b) Verminderung von strahleninduzierten Vitamin-E-und -B_1-Verlusten durch Bestrahlung von Lebensmitteln bei tiefen Temperaturen und durch Ausschluß von Luftsauerstoff. *Zeitschrift für Lebensmittel-Untersuchung und -Forschung*, **169**:276–280.

Diehl JF (1981) Effects of combination processes on the nutritive value of food. In: *Combination processes in food irradiation. Proceedings of a Symposium held in Colombo, Sri Lanka, November 1980.* Vienna, International Atomic Energy Agency, pp. 349–366.

Diehl JF (1990) *Safety of irradiated foods.* New York, Marcel Dekker.

Diehl JF (1991) Nutritional effects of combining irradiation with other treatments. *Food control,* **2**:20–25.

Diehl JF et al. (1991) Regulation of food irradiation in the European Community: Is nutrition an issue? *Food control,* **2**:212–219.

FAO (1962) *Report of the FAO/WHO/IAEA Meeting on the Wholesomeness of Irradiated Foods, Brussels, 23–30 October 1961.* Rome, Food and Agriculture Organization of the United Nations.

FAO (1984) *Codex General Standard for Irradiated Foods and Recommended International Code of Practice for the Operation of Radiation Facilities used for the Treatment of Food.* Rome, Food and Agriculture Organization of the United Nations (CAC/Vol. XV-Ed. 1).

FAO (1991) *Codex General Standard for the Labelling of Prepackaged Foods.* Rome, Food and Agriculture Organization of the United Nations (Codes STAN 1-1985 (Rev. 1-1991)).

Fesus I et al. (1981) Protection of oranges by gamma radiation against *Ceratitis capitata* Wied. *Acta alimentaria,* **10**:293–299.

Forbes AL, Allen MR (1958) *The medical protection plan for the irradiated food taste panel.* US Army Medical Research and Nutrition Laboratory, report no. 221, 17 June 1958 (unpublished document; obtainable in microfiche form from Defense Technical Information Center, DTIC-2DA, Cameron Station, Alexandria, VA 22304–6145, USA).

Galetto W et al. (1979) Irradiation treatment of onion powder: effects on chemical constituents. *Journal of food science,* **44**:591–595.

Hammer CT, Wills FD (1979) The effect of ionizing radiation on the fatty acid composition of natural fats and on lipid peroxide formation. *International journal of radiation biology,* **35**:323–332.

Health and Welfare Canada (1987) *Comprehensive federal government response to report of the standing committee on consumer and corporate affairs on the question of food irradiation and the labelling of irradiated foods.* Ottawa.

IAEA (1989) *Acceptance, control of, and trade in irradiated food.* Vienna, International Atomic Energy Agency.

Janave MT, Thomas P (1979) Influence of post-harvest storage temperature and gamma irradiation on potato carotenoids. *Potato research*, **22**:365–369.

Josephson ES, Peterson MS, eds. (1982) *Preservation of food by ionizing irradiation.* Boca Raton, FL, CRC Press.

Kennedy TS, Ley FJ (1971) Studies on the combined effect of gamma radiation and cooking on the nutritional value of food. *Journal of the science of food and agriculture*, **22**:146–148.

Levy LM et al. (1957) *An assessment of the possible toxic effects to human beings of short-term consumption of food sterilized with gamma rays.* US Army Medical Research and Nutrition Laboratory, Report No. 203, 25 March 1957 (unpublished document; obtainable in microfiche form from Defense Technical Information Center, DTIC-2DA, Cameron Station, Alexandria, VA 22304–6145, USA).

McGary VE et al. (1957) *Acceptability of irradiated food consumed by human subjects.* US Army Medical Research and Nutrition Laboratory, Report No. 200, 15 March 1957 (unpublished document; obtainable in microfiche form from Defense Technical Information Center, DTIC-2DA, Cameron Station, Alexandria, VA 22304–6145, USA).

Mameesh MS et al. (1964) Studies on the radiation preservation of fish. I. The effect on certain vitamins in fresh fillets of cod and dogfish and in smoked fillets of cod and herring. *Reports on technological research concerning Norwegian fish industry*, Vol. IV, No. 10, 10pp.

Ministry of Agriculture (1983). [*Irradiation of foods? Report of an Expert Committee.*] Stockholm (Statens Offentliga Utredninger No. 26) (in Swedish).

Muller H (1991) Bestimmung der Folsäure-Gehalte von Lebensmittein — der Einfluss der Verabeitung auf das Verteilungsmuster. [Determination of folic acid content of foodstuffs—effect of processing on the distribution pattern.] *Ernährungsumschau*, **38**:101.

Murray TK (1983) Nutritional aspects of food irradiation. In: Elias PS, Cohen AJ, eds. *Recent advances in food irradiation.* Amsterdam, Elsevier Biomedical, pp. 203–216.

Nagay NY, Moy JH (1985) Quality of gamma irradiated California Valencia oranges. *Journal of food science*, **50**:215–219.

National Food Agency (1986) *Irradiation of food. Report of a Danish working group.* Søborg (Publication No. 120).

Plough IC et al. (1957) *An evaluation in human beings of the acceptability, digestibility and toxicity of pork sterilized by gamma radiation and stored at room temperatures.* US Army Medical Research and Nutrition Laboratory, Report No. 204, 17 May 1957 (unpublished document; obtainable in microfiche form from Defense Technical Information Center, DTIC-2DA, Cameron Station, Alexandria, VA 22304–6145, USA).

Plough IC et al. (1960) Human feeding studies with irradiated foods. *Federation proceedings,* **19**:1052.

Scientific Committee for Food (1987) *Report on irradiated foods.* Brussels, Commission of the European Communities (Food Science and Techniques Series No. 10840).

Sreenivasan A (1974) Compositional and quality changes in some irradiated foods. In: *Improvement of food quality by irradiation.* Vienna, International Atomic Energy Agency, pp. 129–115.

Thayer DW (1990) Food irradiation: benefits and concerns. *Journal of food quality,* **13**:147–169.

Thomas MH et al. (1981) Effect of irradiation and conventional processing on thiamin content of pork. *Journal of food science,* **46**:824–828.

Tipples KH, Norris FW (1965) Some effects of high levels of gamma irradiation on the lipids of wheat. *Cereal chemistry,* **42**:437–451.

Vaca CE, Harms-Ringdahl M (1986) Radiation-induced lipid peroxidation in whole grain of rye, wheat and rice: effects on linoleic and linolenic acid. *Radiation physics and chemistry,* **28**:325–330.

WHO (1965) *The technical basis for legislation on irradiated food. Report of a Joint FAO/IAEA/WHO Expert Committee.* Geneva, World Health Organization (WHO Technical Report Series, No. 316).

WHO (1970) *Wholesomeness of irradiated food with special reference to wheat, potatoes and onions. Report of a Joint FAO/IAEA/WHO Expert Committee.* Geneva, World Health Organization (WHO Technical Report Series, No. 451).

WHO (1977) *Wholesomeness of irradiated food. Report of a Joint FAO/IAEA/WHO Expert Committee.* Geneva, World Health Organization (WHO Technical Report Series, No. 604).

WHO (1981) *Wholesomeness of irradiated food. Report of a Joint FAO/IAEA/WHO Expert Committee.* Geneva, World Health Organization (WHO Technical Report Series, No. 659).

WHO (1988) *Food irradiation. A technique for preserving and improving the safety of food.* Geneva, World Health Organization.

9.
Concerns and overall conclusions

9.1 Concerns expressed about irradiated food

9.1.1 Conflicting results and conclusions

Concern has been expressed that research on the safety and nutritional adequacy of irradiated food has yielded some conflicting results and conclusions. As explained in Chapters 6 and 8, the vast number of studies undertaken under a myriad of different circumstances were bound, for statistical reasons alone, to produce some conflicting results, but these are remarkably few, and even fewer remain unexplained (see Chapter 6). None of the conflicting results identified constitute reasonable grounds for rejecting the use of irradiated food. It should be recognized that scientific consensus does not depend on every scientist agreeing with certain conclusions, but rather on how the entire body of scientific evidence is interpreted by the scientific community.

9.1.2 Radiolytic substances

Concern has also been expressed about the possibility that the substances formed within food by irradiation (radiolytic substances) may be toxic. As mentioned in Chapter 4, the likelihood of truly unique radiolytic products occurring is low; most of the products identified in irradiated food have also been found in non-irradiated food. Toxicological studies have shown that the radiolytic substances pose no health risks as typically consumed. This extensive body of analytical data, together with the large number of toxicological studies, shows as conclusively as science is capable that irradiation of food produces no substances that would be harmful at the levels consumed.

9.1.3 Fears of radioactive food

Chapters 4 and 5 explain that, with the energy limitations accepted throughout the world (10 MeV for electrons, 5 MeV for X-rays, and 1.33 MeV for cobalt-60), the fear that food will become radioactive is unfounded.

9.1.4 Dead food

There is some concern that food will become "dead" and valueless following irradiation, where the word "dead" in this context means that food such as

SAFETY AND NUTRITIONAL ADEQUACY OF IRRADIATED FOOD

vegetables, for example, which are alive in a biochemical sense, would be rendered lifeless by irradiation. Scientifically (and nutritionally), food value depends solely on the nutritional value of the irradiated food. The effect of irradiation on the nutritional value of food is dealt with in detail in Chapter 8. Murray (1990) raised the additional concern that irradiation may lead to cellular damage to fruits and vegetables, a possibility that is discussed in Chapter 4. It should be noted that, if it were to lead to more rapid spoilage, there would be no incentive to use irradiation with these commodities.

9.1.5 Use of irradiation to restore contaminated food

The possibility that irradiation may be used to "clean up" food that is unacceptably contaminated is another concern that has been expressed from time to time. While what is meant by "unacceptably contaminated" is not explicitly defined, it is assumed that the reference is to microbiological contamination and the possibility that attempts might be made to use irradiation to improve the appearance of spoiled food. However, radiation is not capable of restoring the appearance or normal organoleptic characteristics of spoiled food. It may destroy the microorganisms present in food, as described in Chapter 7, but it cannot destroy off-odours, off-tastes or the off-appearance of spoiled food. There is, therefore, no basis for the concern that irradiation may be used for the restoration and marketing of spoiled food.

9.1.6 Aflatoxin

It has been suggested that aflatoxin-producing moulds may thrive in irradiated food, a concern addressed and discussed in Chapter 7, where it is concluded that the available scientific data indicate that food irradiated and stored under typical conditions would be at no increased risk of aflatoxin production. Experiments that did indicate increased aflatoxin production after irradiation were carried out under laboratory conditions not conceivable in practice.

9.1.7 Botulism

As described in Chapter 7, the undetected growth of *Clostridium botulinum* has been the subject of a number of studies on chicken and fish. It has been amply demonstrated that irradiation presents no unique or unusual problems beyond those encountered in many other nonsterilizing food processes. This means that adequate precautions must be taken to ensure that processed foods that could support the growth of *C. botulinum* are stored under appropriate conditions. For example, it is recommended that irradiated fish be stored at temperatures of 3 °C or lower to ensure the absence of toxin throughout the storage life.

9. CONCERNS AND OVERALL CONCLUSIONS

9.1.8 Nutrients

Chapter 8 explicitly addresses nutritional concerns, and it is concluded that the possible adverse effects of food irradiation on human nutritional well-being will be of a similar magnitude as those of other forms of food preservation.

9.1.9 Resistant microorganisms

As discussed in Chapter 7, the large body of scientific knowledge concerning radiation-resistant microorganisms indicates that such microorganisms, whether a product of selection or mutation, would be less robust than typical wild-type microorganisms in the normal environment. Consequently, it is considered that such organisms would typically be lost and would not reappear in other foods undergoing irradiation. The analogy with heat-resistant microorganisms was discussed in the same chapter and it was pointed out that such microorganisms have not given rise to problems in thermal processing and that there is no reason to believe that radiation-resistant organisms would cause problems in food irradiation.

9.1.10 Organoleptic effects

There is some concern that food irradiation may have deleterious effects on taste, smell and texture. Irradiation can certainly damage the organoleptic quality of food if improperly or inappropriately applied. Given the adverse consequences that such effects would have on consumer acceptability, it seems unlikely that they would cause problems for the consumer. Instead, the consumer would be expected to insist on the high quality which, as described in Chapters 3 and 8, is achievable with irradiated food.

9.1.11 Labelling

The possibility that labelling requirements will not be enforced and that the consumer will therefore not have a choice has been cited as an objection to food irradiation. Labelling a food as having been irradiated is no different from labelling a dairy product as having been pasteurized. Such labelling is undertaken both because it is required by law and because this form of processing is viewed positively by the consumer. In the case of fruits and vegetables, irradiation prolongs storage life; in the case of fish and meat, it destroys harmful pathogens. The retailer of irradiated food would usually want the consumer to know that the food has this additional advantage. It is likely that labels declaring that food has been irradiated would be required by law and there is no reason to suppose that such labelling requirements would be ignored by government authorities.

9.1.12 Lack of adequate controls

This concern relates solely to international trade and has not been explicitly addressed here, although it is covered by implication in Chapters 3, 5 and 8. It is considered highly unlikely that any irradiated food would be imported from countries that do not apply the Codex General Standard for Irradiated Food and the Recommended International Code of Practice for the Operation of Irradiation Facilities used for the Treatment of Food, as adopted by the Codex Alimentarius Commission. The rapidly improving post-irradiation detection methods, as described in Chapter 5, will help to ascertain this.

9.1.13 Dose uniformity

It has been suggested that there may be a lack of dose uniformity, especially in large boxes where some foods will receive higher doses. This is a technical matter for the irradiation facility and is covered by the specific protocols designed to limit the maximum level of radiation for any food in any configuration. In countries where food irradiation is permitted, such protocols have been laid down, and adherence to them is enforced by inspection authorities.

9.1.14 Post-irradiation detection methodology

Intensive studies with the aim of developing tests to determine whether food has been irradiated were described in Chapter 5. Although no single generic test for qualitatively and quantitatively assessing irradiation in food is likely to become available in the near future, useful post-irradiation detection methods for specific foods have been developed for regulatory and surveillance purposes. The practical usefulness of these tests can only be examined once foods have been approved for irradiation under specified conditions, and irradiated products have entered trade.

9.1.15 Re-irradiation

The possibility that food could be re-irradiated has been suggested. It should be noted that the Codex General Standard for Irradiated Foods (FAO, 1984) allows food with low moisture content, e.g. cereals, pulses, and dehydrated food, to be re-irradiated for the purpose of controlling insect infestation. Re-irradiation of such products is comparable to re-fumigation, which is commonly practised by the food industry and trade for the same purpose.

The same Codex Standard prohibits re-irradiation of other foods. Provided that food irradiation is conducted in accordance with good manufacturing practice in properly licensed, supervised and inspected plants, this seems as unlikely as food being repasteurized. Even if good manufacturing practice were to be disregarded, it is hard to imagine a toxicological, microbiological or nutritional risk arising from occasional re-irradiation.

9.2 Overall conclusions

Irradiated food produced in accordance with established good manufacturing practice can be considered safe and nutritionally adequate because the process of irradiation:

- will not lead to changes in the composition of the food that, from a toxicological point of view, would have an adverse effect on human health;
- will not lead to changes in the microflora of the food that would increase the microbiological risk to the consumer;
- will not lead to nutrient losses to an extent that would have an adverse effect on the nutritional status of individuals or populations.

References

FAO (1984) *Codex General Standard for Irradiated Foods*. Rome, Food and Agriculture Organization of the United Nations (Codex Alimentarius, Vol. XV).

Murray DR (1990) *Biology of food irradiation*. New York, John Wiley.

Annex
Participants in WHO Consultation on Food Irradiation
Geneva, 20–22 May 1992

Experts*

Professor J.F. Diehl, Director and Professor, Bundesforschungsanstalt für Ernährung, Karlsruhe, Germany

Dr W.G. Flamm, Flamm Associates, Reston, VA, USA

Dr A.L. Forbes, Medical Consultant and Chairman, International Union of Nutritional Sciences Committee on the Nutritional Aspects of Food Standards, Rockville, MD, USA

Dr I. Knudsen, Head, Toksikologisk Institut, Ministry of Health, National Food Agency, Søborg, Denmark

Professor B.E.B. Moseley, Head of Laboratory, Agricultural and Food Research Council's Institute of Food Research, Reading Laboratory, Reading, England (*Chairman*)

Dr G.H. Pauli, Chief, Novel Ingredients and Food, Division of Food and Color Additives, Office of Compliance, Center for Food Safety and Applied Nutrition, US Food and Drug Administration, Washington, DC, USA

Observers

International Consultative Group on Food Irradiation (ICGFI),
Mr M. Satin, FAO Joint Secretary, ICGFI, Chief, Agricultural Services, Food and Agriculture Organization of the United Nations, Rome, Italy

International Organization of Consumers Unions (IOCU)
Dr J. Beishon, Consumers' Association Limited, London, England

National Cancer Institute
Dr D. Langfellow, Chief, Chemical and Physical Carcinogenesis, Division of Cancer Etiology, Bethesda, MD, USA

National Food Authority of Australia
Ms L. Onyon, Acting Scientific Director, Canberra, Australia

---

*Unable to attend: Dr W.W. Nichols, Executive Director, Genetic and Cellular Toxicology, Merck Research Laboratories, Green Lane, PA, USA.

Secretariat*

Dr T. Fujikura, Scientist, Veterinary Public Health, Division of Communicable Diseases, WHO, Geneva, Switzerland

Dr F. Käferstein, Chief, Food Safety, Division of Health Protection and Promotion, WHO, Geneva, Switzerland (*Secretary*)

Dr G. Moy, Scientist, Food Safety, Division of Health Protection and Promotion, WHO, Geneva, Switzerland

Dr J. Rochon, Director, Division of Health Protection and Promotion, WHO, Geneva, Switzerland

---

* A representative of the Programme for the Promotion of Chemical Safety was invited but was unable to attend.

Index

ADMIT (Analytical Detection Methods for Irradiation Treatment of Foods) 51–52
Advisory Committee on Irradiated and Novel Foods 35, 133
Aerobic plate count (APC) 66, 67
Aeromonas hydrophila 122
Aflatoxin xiv, 127–128, 150
Alanine aminotransferase, serum 84, 85
Ames mutagenicity test 101, 102, 104
Amino acids x, 40–41
Anaemia 84–86
Anaerobic conditions 8, 38, 141
Animal products 24–27, 81
Animal studies *see* Toxicity studies
Antimetabolites 142–143
Applications of food irradiation ix–x, 16–28
Ascorbic acid *see* Vitamin C
Aspartate aminotransferase, serum 84, 85
Aspergillus flavus 127
Aspergillus ochraceus 127
Aspergillus parasiticus 127
Association of Official Analytical Chemists (AOAC) 52, 56
Atomic Energy Commission, USA 5
Avocados 21

Background radiation 35–36
Bacteria
    radiation-resistant 10–11, 126–127, 151
    radiation sensitivity 10, 122–123
Beef x, 25, 43–44
Beef tapeworm x, 25
Biotin 142

Bone marrow cells 95–101
Botulism 123–125, 150
Brucella abortus 122
Brynjolfsson formula 9
Bulbs 61
2,3–Butanediol 58

Caesium–137 6
Campylobacter x, 24
Campylobacter jejuni 122
Canada 133
Canning 4
Carbohydrates
    chemical changes x, 8, 39–40
    detection of radiolytic products 56–57
    nutritional value xiv, 138
Carbon dioxide treatment 27
Carbonyl compounds 56
Carcinogenicity studies 89–94, 102–103
Carotene 140, 141
Carotenoids 141
Central Institute for Nutrition and Food Research (Netherlands) xiii, 104–105
Chemical treatments 18, 27
Chemiluminescence (CL) 63–64, 65
Chemistry, irradiation (*see also* Radiolytic products) x–xi, 35–45
Chicken *see* Poultry
China, human toxicity studies 103–104
Chromosomal abnormalities 96–98, 99–101
Citrus fruits 60–61, 65

Clostridium botulinum xiii, 26, 123–125, 150
  type E 26, 123
  types A and B 124
Clostridium perfringens 24, 25
Cobalamin 139
Cobalt-60 6
Codex Alimentarius Commission 2, 12, 35, 128
Codex Committee on Methods of Analysis and Sampling 52
Codex General Standard for Irradiated Foods 2, 12
Community Bureau of Reference of the Commission of the European Communities (BCR) 51, 52, 67
Concerns 2, 149–153
Cooking 136, 137
Cyanocobalamin (vitamin B_{12}) 139, 142
Cyclobutanones 56
Cysticercosis x, 25

D_{10} values 10, 122
"Dead" food 149–150
Decay, prevention of 21–22
Dehydration 5
Deinococcus radiodurans 10–11
Denmark 133
Detection, post-irradiation xii, 50–67, 152
  harmonization of protocols and testing strategies 66–67
  international activities 51–52
  methods 52–66
    chemical changes 52–58
    histological and morphological effects 65
    microflora 66
    physical properties 58–65
Differential scanning calorimetry (DSC) 60
Dilution effect 38
Direct epifluorescent filter technique (DEFT) 66, 67
DNA
  detection of damage 57, 67
  effects of radiation 9–10

Dose (radiation) 36, 122–123
  high 17, 132
  inactivation 10
  low 17, 132
  maximum permissible 35
  mean lethal (MLD) 10
  medium 17, 132
  nutritional quality and 136
  radiolytic products and 43
  required to kill 90% (D_{10}) 10, 122
  toxicity studies 106
  uniformity 152
Drosophila melanogaster 101, 102
Dry foods (*see also* Spices) x, 22–23
  detection of irradiated 64
  fruits and vegetables 22

Eggs 27
Electrical impedance 59
Electron beams 35
  generators 6–7
  grain irradiation 23
  maximum permissible dose 35
  nutritional losses and 136
Electron spin resonance (ESR) 60–63, 67
Electrons, low-energy solvated 37
Embryo test 65
Enzyme-linked immunosorbent assay (ELISA) 57
Enzymes 40
Escherichia coli 25, 122, 126
Ethanol 58
Ethoxyquin 105
Ethylene oxide 23
European Communities, Commission of 134

Fats *see* Lipids
Fatty acids, polyunsaturated 138
Federation of American Societies for Experimental Biology 44
Fish 26–27
  control of pathogens 124–125
  detection of irradiated 62–63
Folic acid 139, 142
Food
  as multicomponent system 38

INDEX

Food (*continued*)
   contaminated 150
   "dead" 149–150
   organoleptic quality 151
Food and Agriculture Organization of the United Nations (FAO) 1, 2, 11–13
Food and Drug Administration (FDA) 35, 123, 133
   database of toxicity studies 82–102
Food irradiation 4–13
   applications ix–x, 16–28
   chemistry x–xi, 35–45
   combination processes 27–28
   concerns about 2, 149–153
   functions 17
   international controls 152–153
   mechanism 7–9
   overall conclusions 153
   previous reviews 11–13
   process 7
   repeated 152–153
Food preservation 1, 4–5
   combination processes 27–28
Foodborne disease 4, 122–123
Free radicals 8, 36–37, 52
   chemical reactivity 9, 37
   detection 60
Frozen food 8, 39, 137
Fruit
   dried 22
   fresh ix, 18–22
   composition and quality 21
   detection of irradiated 60–61, 65
   radiation sensitivity 20

Gamma radiation 6, 36, 38
Gas-liquid chromatography (GLC) 56, 58
Glucose 39–40, 101
Grains/grain products 23, 61
Grapes 61
Gray (Gy) 9
Growth
   animals fed irradiated food 84, 89, 92
   differential 123–125
   inhibition of 18–19

Haemorrhagic diathesis 84
Heart lesions 92–93
Heat treatment 28, 136, 137
Helminths, parasitic 11, 25, 26
Hepatitis A virus 10, 26
Herbs 22, 63
Hexadecadiene xi, 44
Histological effects 65
Hydration *see* Water content
Hydrocarbons 55–56
Hydrogen 37
   detection 58
Hydrogen peroxide 37, 38
Hydroperoxy radical 38
Hydroxyl radicals 8, 37

Impedance, electrical 59
Insect disinfestation ix, 11, 19, 23
International Atomic Energy Agency (IAEA) 1, 11–13, 51
International Committee on Food Microbiology and Hygiene (ICFMH) 12, 128
International Document on Food Irradiation 12–13
International Organization for Standardization (ISO) 52
International Project in the Field of Food Irradiation (IFIP) xii–xiii, 1, 105
International Union of Pure and Applied Chemistry (IUPAC) 51, 52
Irradiated Foods Task Force 133

Joint FAO/IAEA/WHO Expert Committee on the Wholesomeness of Irradiated Food 1–2, 106
   activities 11–12
   dose recommendations 35–36
   nutritional quality and 133

Labelling 143, 151
Lipids (fats)
   chemical changes x–xi, 9, 41–42
   detection of radiolytic products 55–56
   irradiated meat 41–42, 43
   nutritional value xiv, 138
   unique radiolytic products 44–45

Listeria 24, 125
Luminescence 63–65
Lymphocytes, peripheral 101

Macronutrients (*see also* Carbohydrates; Lipids; Proteins) 81
  chemical changes x–xi, 8–9, 39–42
  detection of radiolytic products 52–57
  nutritional value xiv, 138
Malnourished children, polyploidy in xiii, 94–95
Malonaldehyde 56
Mean lethal dose (MLD) 10
Meat ix, 24–25
  detection of irradiated 61–62, 66
  radiolytic products 41–42, 43–44
Microbiology xiii–xiv, 122–128
Micrococcus radiodurans 10–11
Microorganisms (*see also* Bacteria)
  irradiated foods 66
  mutations in xiv, 11, 125–127
  radiation-resistant 10–11, 126–127, 151
  selective killing and differential growth 123–125
  toxin production 10, 127–128
Milk pasteurization 2, 4–5
Minerals xv, 139
Moraxella acinetobacter 10–11
Morphological effects 65
Moulds 10
Mushrooms ix, 21, 65
Mussels 62–63
Mutagenicity studies 94–102
Mutations
  dominant lethal 94, 96–98, 102
  in microorganisms xiv, 11, 125–127
Mycotoxins 10, 127–128

Near-infrared analysis (NIR) 60
Nicotinic acid (niacin)
  factors affecting losses 136, 137, 141, 142
  radiation sensitivity 42, 139, 140
Nucleic acids 9, 57
Nutritional quality (*see also* Macronutrients; Vitamins; *specific nutrients*) xiv–xv, 132–145, 151

Nutritional quality (*continued*)
  conflicting research 149
  dietary role of irradiated food and 143
  factors affecting 135–138, 141–142
  fruits and vegetables 21
  labelling and 143
  postmarketing surveillance 144
  preregistration requirements 143
  research needs 144
  synopsis of reviews 133–135
Nuts 22

Ochratoxin 127
Onions 19, 65
Organoleptic effects 151
Oxygen
  irradiation chemistry and 8, 38
  vitamin losses and 140

Pantothenic acid 142
Paprika 22, 138
Parasitic helminths 11, 25, 26
Pasteurization 2, 4–5
Pathogenicity, increased 10–11, 125–126
Pentadecadiene xi, 44
Pest control ix, 11, 19, 23–24
Pesticides 19, 23
pH effects 39
Phenylalanine 55
Plant products 18–24, 81
Polyploidy 94–101
  human studies in China 103–104
  in malnourished children xiii, 94–95
Polyunsaturated fatty acids 138
Pork x, 25, 55
Post-irradiation detection *see* Detection, post-irradiation
Postmarketing surveillance 144
Potatoes 18, 59, 65, 66
Poultry ix, x, 24
  control of pathogens 123–124
  detection of irradiated 62
Preregistration requirements 143
Preservation of food *see* Food preservation
Protein efficiency ratio (PER) 138

INDEX

Proteins
  chemical changes x, 8–9, 40–41
  detection of radiolytic products
    54–55
  nutritional value xiv, 138
Proteus vulgaris 122
Protons, hydrated 37
Protozoa 11
Pseudomonas fluorescens 122
Pyridoxine (vitamin B_6) 84, 139, 142

Radappertization 16
Radiation
  activity in biological systems 9–11
  background 35–36
  dose *see* Dose (radiation)
  ionizing x, 36
  primary effects 8, 36–37
  resistance 10–11, 125–127, 151
  secondary effects 8, 37
  sources 5–7, 136
  types 36
Radicidation 16
Radioactivity, induced xi–xii, 7, 35–36, 149
Radiolysis 8
Radiolytic products x–xi, 8–9, 36–37
  concerns about 149
  detection methods 52–66
  factors affecting 8, 37–39
  total yield 43
  toxicology *see* Toxicity studies
  unique xi, 43–45
Radurization 17
Raltech xii–xiii, 102–103
Re-irradiation 152
Refrigeration 4, 28
Reproduction studies 87–89
Riboflavin
  factors affecting losses 137, 142
  radiation sensitivity 42, 139, 140
Ripening, delay of ix, 20–21

Salmonella xiii
  eggs 27
  poultry x, 24
  seafood 25
Salmonella anatum 122

Salmonella enteritidis 122
Salmonella newport 122
Salmonella typhimurium 126
Seafood 25–26
  detection of irradiated 62–63, 66
Senescence, delay of 20–21
Shelf-life, extension of ix, 122–123
Shellfish 26, 62–63
Shigella 26, 122
Shrimps 26, 27, 56, 59, 63
Spices x, 22–23
  detection of irradiated 58, 59–60, 63, 64–65
Sprouting, inhibition of ix, 18–19
Staphylococcus 24, 25
Starch 40
Storage conditions, nutrient losses and 141–142
Strawberries ix, 21–22
  detection of irradiated 60–61, 65, 66
Subchronic toxicity studies 84–86, 104
Sweden 133
Sweet potatoes 18–19

Temperature (*see also* Frozen food)
  irradiation chemistry and 39
  nutrient losses and xv, 136–137
  storage of potatoes 18
Teratology studies 87–89, 102
Testicular tumours 102–103
Thermal analysis 60
Thermoluminescence (TL) 63, 64–65, 67
Thiamine (vitamin B_1)
  as marker of irradiation 58
  factors affecting losses 136, 137–138, 142
  radiation sensitivity 42, 139, 140
Thymine glycol 57
Thyroiditis 93
α-Tocopherol (vitamin E) 42, 137, 140, 141, 142
Toxicity studies 81–105
  chronic 89–94, 102–103, 104–105
  conflicting research 149
  in FDA database 82–102

Toxicity studies (*continued*)
 human feeding, in China 103–104
 mutagenesis 94–102
 Raltech 102–103
 reproduction and teratology studies 87–89, 102
 subchronic 84–86, 104
Toxicology xii–xiii, 81–107
Toxins, bacterial 10
Toxoplasma gondii 25
Trace elements xv
Trichinella spiralis x, 25
Triglycerides 41
o-Tyrosine 55

Undecyne xi, 44
United Kingdom 133
United States of America 133
United States Army 5, 25, 43, 132, 133

Vacuum packaging 28
Vegetables
 composition and quality 21
 detection of irradiated 65–66
 fresh ix, 18–22
 radiation sensitivity 20
Vibrio cholerae 26
Vibrio parahaemolyticus 26, 122
Virulence, increased 10–11, 125–126
Viruses 10–11
Viscosity 57, 59–60
Vitamin A 140–141, 142
Vitamin B_1 *see* Thiamine
Vitamin B_6 (pyridoxine) 84, 139, 142
Vitamin B_{12} (cyanocobalamin) 139, 142

Vitamin C (ascorbic acid)
 factors affecting losses 138, 142
 radiation sensitivity 42, 139–140
Vitamin D 140, 141, 142
Vitamin E (α-tocopherol) 42, 137, 140, 142
Vitamin K 84, 140, 141, 142
Vitamins (*see also specific vitamins*)
 detection of radiolytic products 57–58
 factors affecting losses 141–143
 fat-soluble 140–141
 radiation sensitivity xi, xiv, 42, 139–141
 significance of losses 143
 water-soluble 139–140
Volatile chemicals xi, 41, 44
 detection 55–56, 58

Water content (hydration)
 irradiation chemistry and x, 37–38
 nutritional losses and 137–138
 reducing 28
Wheat, ingestion of irradiated xiii, 94–101
World Health Organization (WHO) 1, 2, 11–13, 51

X-rays 36
 generators 6–7
 maximum permissible dose 35

Yams 19
Yeasts 10
Yersinia 24, 26, 122, 125

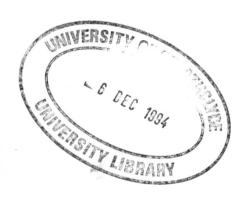